Intimate Partner Abuse and Health Professionals

Commissioning Editor: Susan Young
Development Editor: Catherine Jackson
Project Manager: Cheryl Brant
Designer: Stewart Larking

Intimate Partner Abuse and Health Professionals: New Approaches to Domestic Violence

Edited by

Gwenneth Roberts PhD BBus(Health Admin) RN

...ment of Psychiatry, University of Queensland, Brisbane,

BBS FRACGP DRANZCOG PhD

...neral Practice, University of Melbourne, Carlton, Victoria, Australia

GP

...nd Development, Centre for General Practice and Primary Care,
...School of Medicine and Dentistry, London, UK

OXFORD PHILADELPHIA ST LOUIS SYDNEY TORONTO 2006

CHURCHILL
LIVINGSTONE
ELSEVIER

First published 2006

ISBN 0 443 07493 3

British Library Cataloguing in Publication Data
A catalogue record for this book is available from the British Library

Library of Congress Cataloging in Publication Data
A catalog record for this book is available from the Library of Congress

Notice
Knowledge and best practice in this field are constantly changing. As new research and experience broaden our knowledge, changes in practice, treatment and drug therapy may become necessary or appropriate. Readers are advised to check the most current information provided (i) on procedures featured or (ii) by the manufacturer of each product to be administered, to verify the recommended dose or formula, the method and duration of administration, and contraindications. It is the responsibility of the practitioner, relying on their own experience and knowledge of the patient, to make diagnoses, to determine dosages and the best treatment for each individual patient, and to take all appropriate safety precautions. To the fullest extent of the law, neither the publisher nor the authors nor editors assume any liability for any injury and/or damage.

The Publisher

Printed in Italy

Contents

SECTION 1 – History and background issues

Chapter 1

Chapter 2

SECTION 2 – Impact, education, identification, and intervention

Chapter 3

Chapter 4

Chapter 5

Chapter 6

Contributors

Judy Atkinson PhD
*Director, College of Indigenous Australian Peoples,
Southern Cross University, Lismore, New South
Wales, Australia*

Jacquelyn C Campbell PhD RN FAAN
*Anna D. Wolf Chair, Associate Dean for Faculty
Affairs, Johns Hopkins University School of Nursing,
Baltimore, Maryland, USA*

Gene Feder MD FRCGP
*Professor of Primary Care Research and
Development, Centre for General Practice and
Primary Care, Barts and the London, Queen Mary's
School of Medicine and Dentistry, London, UK*

Nancy Glass PhD MPH RN
*Co-Director, Center for Health Disparities Research,
Assistant Professor, Oregon Health and Science
University, School of Nursing, Portland, Oregon,
USA*

Kelsey Hegarty PhD MBBS FRACGP DRANZCOG
*Associate Professor, Department of General Practice,
University of Melbourne, Carlton, Victoria,
Australia*

Kathryn Laughon PhD RN
*Assistant Professor, University of Virginia School of
Nursing, Charlottesville, Virginia, USA*

Heather McCosker-Howard PhD RN RM
BAppSci(Nsg) MNsg GradCertEd(Tertiary Ed)
*Lecturer, School of Nursing, Queensland
University of Technology, Brisbane, Queensland,
Australia*

Jean Ramsay PhD
*Senior Research Officer, Centre for General Practice
and Primary Care, Barts and the London, Queen
Mary's School of Medicine and Dentistry, London,
UK*

Michael V Relf PhD APRN BC AACRN CCRN
*Assistant Professor and Chair, Department of
Professional Nursing, Georgetown University, School
of Nursing and Health Studies, Washington, DC,
USA*

Gwenneth Roberts PhD BBus(Health Admin) RN
*Honorary Research Consultant, Department of
Psychiatry, University of Queensland, Brisbane,
Queensland, Australia*

Michael A Rodríguez MD MPH
*Associate Professor, David Geffen School of Medicine
at University College of Los Angeles, Department of
Family Medicine, Los Angeles, California, USA*

George Saba PhD
*Professor of Clinical Family and Community
Medicine, Family and Community Medicine,
University of California, San Francisco, California,
USA*

Jocelynne Scutt MA LLB LLM LLU SJD LLD
DipJuris DipLegalStudies CCA ACCA
*Barrister and Film-maker/Executive Producer, Health
Complaints Conciliator New South Wales, Australia*

Judy Shakespeare MA BM BCh MRCP FRCGP
*General Practitioner and Research Associate,
National Perinatal Epidemiology Unit, Institute of
Health Sciences, Oxford, UK*

Jennifer Smith PhD M Soc Wk Bn Soc Wk
Senior Lecturer, School of Social Work and Applied Human Sciences, University of Queensland, Brisbane, Australia

Angela Taft MPH PhD
Research Fellow, Mother and Child Health Research, La Trobe University, Carlton, Victoria, Australia

Carole Warshaw MD
Department of Medicine, John H. Stroger Jr Hospital of Cook County, Director, Domestic Violence and Mental Health Policy Initiative, Chicago, Illinois, USA

Anne B Woods PhD RN CNM
Assistant Professor, Johns Hopkins University School of Nursing, Baltimore, Maryland, USA

Mary Zachary MD MS
Assistant Professor of Family and Social Medicine, Montefiore Medical Center, Albert Einstein College of Medicine of Yeshiva University, New York, USA

Foreword

Beverley Raphael

A SCHOLARLY AND COMPASSIONATE TEXT

This excellent volume sets a very high standard of scholarship in exploring and reviewing the field of intimate partner violence and its relevance for health and health care professionals. The editors, both in their own contributions and through the contributions of their selected authors, have gathered the current scientific and clinical basis that is essential to addressing this problem. The work is thoughtful, thorough, compassionate and positive in its approach. The themes are held consistently through Gwenneth Roberts' historical overview of this 'old' problem and its acknowledgement in recent decades; Kelsey Hegarty's synthesis of the epidemiology building on definitional problems, theories of causation, measurement complexities, and the range of studies and data sets from which information can be drawn. This critical background information leads into the following section which deals with impacts, education, identification, and intervention. The literature makes clear the profound impacts on women's mental and physical health, on their pregnancies and childbearing, and on their children of all ages and into the next generation. Nevertheless ongoing societal and personal attitudes, the need for education and training at the most basic as well as sophisticated levels, and the complexities of translating what is known into effective clinical practice means there is still a great deal to be done to impact on this problem. Indeed these complexities are even more profound when considered in the context of the whole family, and how to respond. This is the more so because of the limited research

base to inform clinical and other intervention, although there are hopeful indications for the roles of social advocacy and clinical interventions in Cognitive Behavior Therapy and group modalities.

A particular issue is how to create institutional and structural change that can effectively address the multiple social, cultural, and personal determinants. The emphasis on an integrated ecological model suggests a valuable, if complex, theoretical basis that can inform both research and practice. That clinical practice alone is insufficient is highlighted by all authors and made perhaps more obvious by Jocelynne Scutt's analysis of the medico-legal issues 'Medico-legal issues: when women speak into silence' (Chapter 10).

The role of a public health, or a new public health approach is highlighted in a number of ways. Gene Feder *et al.* ('Clinical response to women experiencing intimate partner abuse: what is the evidence for good practice and policy', Chapter 6) highlight the scientific and clinical debates about the evidence base for screening in health care settings, and the limitations of the evidence currently available to inform good practice and policy. These authors review available guidelines for practice in terms of prevention, screening, primary care, and health care settings generally, but emphasize the primacy of safety; first not to harm; and recognizing always the need to not place the woman or her children at greater risk. Public health impacts are also relevant in terms of the health burden on children (Jennifer Smith, 'What is the impact of intimate partner abuse on children?' Chapter 8) and also on childbearing women for the physical and mental health effects, including risk not only of increased morbidity, but mortality. A recent 'burden of disease' study has highlighted the massive contribution of domestic violence in the population health contexts. Most clearly, however Judy Atkinson ('Intimate partner abuse and indigenous people', Chapter 12) reviews the profound impacts of family violence for indigenous peoples, its origins in colonization trauma and loss, and the need to see interventions from a new public health approach taking into account ecological, historical, community, cultural, and clinical themes to lessen its profound impact in such settings.

Cultural issues as they relate to the status and place of women remain a central issue. This is most obvious when a cultural competency model allows the clinician to understand his or her own cultural values, while at the same time assessing and responding to the violence issues and their implications in different ethnic and cultural groups. Language and other barriers to access also need to be taken into account also. Cultural and attitudinal barriers may also be reflected in homophobia and difficulties in recognizing and responding to intimate partner abuse in gay and lesbian settings, or when women are violent.

In their synthesis of the way forward, Hegarty, Feder, and Roberts ('Intimate partner abuse research and training: the way forward', Chapter 14) highlight the vital importance of advancing our knowledge base through research, education, and training. They also highlight the importance of analysis of the complex processes that contribute to sustaining this age old problem so that it may be prevented and so that when it does present it is asked about and responded to appropriately and effectively in health care as well as other settings.

This scholarly text will set a fine baseline for the future. It is comprehensive, scientifically strong, and a powerful voice for us to do better and to move (as suggested by Judy Atkinson) through the stories of experiences, and experiences shared, sadnesses grieved, fears confronted, safety found, to resilience and ultimately resonance: the capacity for 'growth and the ability to build nurturing respectful relationships' (p. 200).

Beverley Raphael
Professor, Population Mental Health
University of Western Sydney
New South Wales

Foreword

Iona Heath

Human beings suffer, have always suffered and will always suffer: firstly because of the certainty of death and then because of the implacability of nature. Beyond this, not content with the irreducible quota of the inevitable, human beings inflict suffering on each other through violence and other forms of deliberate cruelty and abuse and this, simply because it is not inevitable, is perhaps the most tragic aspect of human suffering.

It is only possible to inflict harm deliberately on another person if one is able to see the other as different and inferior and deserving of hurt. Armies educate soldiers in just this kind of perception. Those who abuse others must first blind themselves to the full subjectivity and dignity of the one they hurt and it is this blinding that makes abuse within intimate relationships so shocking and so painful. Intimate relationships need to be built on love and trust and full recognition and acceptance of the other and all this is betrayed by abuse. No wonder the consequences are so devastating for the future health of the one who is abused and for children who grow up aware of abuse or witnessing it or participating in it.

The great strength of this book is how careful it is to acknowledge and explore the full complexity and difficulty of the challenge posed to health professionals by the existence of intimate partner abuse. The authors never offer simplistic solutions and never extrapolate beyond the research evidence. They are consistently wary of standardized recommendations intended to cover the complexity of every individual situation and they draw attention to the gaps in our understanding, the lack of research in many areas, and the potential harm of ill-considered interventions.

In the consulting room, faced every day with the stories of those struggling to survive within abusive relationships, one of the few reasons to feel optimistic for the future is the commitment and ability of the researchers, so well represented in this book, who are actively engaged in furthering our understanding and helping us all to find ways forward.

Iona Heath
General Practitioner, London

To the mothers of Gwenneth (Lilian Collins), Kelsey (Valda Hegarty),
and Gene (Marika Feder) who encouraged us to become who we are

Preface

Gwenneth Roberts, Kelsey Hegarty, and Gene Feder

This book brings together new information for health professionals about intimate partner abuse (IPA) with a re-thinking of assumptions about how IPA should be addressed in health care settings. This includes tackling issues such as screening, mandatory reporting, understanding abuse in gay and lesbian relationships, and the cultural context of abuse. It will be of value to practitioners, researchers, teachers, and students. The chapters are based on recent research and have been written by international practitioners and researchers from a range of health disciplines. The principles of identification of women experiencing IPA and their assistance by all health professionals are universal. However, this book focuses largely on evidence and policy from Western societies rather than from developing countries.

In response to their own experience and research, this book was conceived by Gwenneth Roberts, an epidemiologist and registered nurse, and Kelsey Hegarty, a social scientist and general practitioner, who observed the failure of many health professionals to identify and assist those who experienced IPA. Gwenneth's observations were made as a result of her research conducted with women and men who presented to the emergency department of a major public hospital in Australia. These studies, the first conducted in an Australian emergency department, revealed that one in five women had a lifetime history of IPA. Her prospective studies (1995 to 1997) revealed much higher rates of depression, anxiety and post-traumatic stress disorder for women who experi-enced IPA than for women who did not have this experience.

Kelsey's interest in the area began when she realized that as a doctor she must be missing many women who had experienced IPA. She embarked on a research programme that looked at developing better measures for IPA to describe women's experience of emotional, physical and sexual abuse (Composite Abuse Scale), their barriers to disclosing such abuse to general practitioners and the high prevalence that existed in women attending Australian general practitioners. Her recent work has also highlighted the close associations with depression and other common presentations in clinical practice.

Five years ago, sitting in a beach house on an island off the coast of Brisbane, Australia, Gwenneth and Kelsey sketched an outline of a book that they believed would provide important information to meet the needs of health professionals on this topic. By 2002 they had assembled a group of international contributors, experienced practition-ers and researchers from a range of disciplines within health care.

It was at this point that Gene Feder joined as a co-editor. A general practitioner in an inner city practice and a primary care researcher, his involvement in developing health service responses to IPA started with the realization that he had not recognized the abuse experienced by some of his women patients and had not responded appropriately to some women who had disclosed abuse. IPA became a major research commitment after his study in east London general practices, showing that almost one-fifth of women consulting their doctors had experienced sexual or physical abuse from a partner in the past year, and two-fifths in their lifetime. He is currently piloting an intervention to improve the response of primary care to women experiencing abuse and is systematically reviewing quantitative and qualitative research on IPA and health services.

Our combined experience and research has shown us that there are many forms of abuse within families and intimate relationships. However, we have chosen to focus on IPA, which includes married and unmarried couples, boyfriends and girlfriends in heterosexual relationships, and lesbian and gay relationships. In this book, the focus will be on partner abuse against women, although we recognize that men can also experience abuse. As the World Health Organization has recently documented, the overwhelming health burden of partner violence is borne by women at the hands of men.[1] However, other issues relating to IPA will be discussed in various chapters, such as the impact on children where adult partners are abusive to one another; and IPA in homosexual relationships. Some issues will be considered in a family context: the management of male partners who perpetrate abuse, women who abuse children, and children who abuse parents. One chapter is devoted entirely to IPA amongst Indigenous peoples. The book will occasionally use the term 'victim' for those who have suffered abuse although we recognize that 'survivor' is an alternative and preferred term by some who have suffered abuse. Still others prefer to speak of having 'experienced' IPA.

This book does not address primary prevention such as community awareness programmes. Preventing the onset of abuse is a large political and cultural challenge to which health services do not directly contribute, other than reflecting the unacceptability of IPA and helping make it a visible problem.

There are three sections to the book: (1) History and background issues; (2) Impact, education, identification, and intervention; (3) Cultural diversity and IPA.

SECTION 1: HISTORY AND BACKGROUND ISSUES

IPA is an ancient problem. Over the last two decades research has demonstrated the high prevalence, and the physical and psychological consequences associated with the problem that bring survivors into contact with the health system. However, failure to identify and assist those who experience IPA appropriately in these settings necessitates new ways of addressing these issues and disseminating the information to health professionals; hence the phrase 'new approaches' in the title. Chapter 1 sets the scene for the chapters that follow. Gwenneth Roberts gives a brief historical overview of IPA as an issue of public concern since the nineteenth century. This historical approach is linked with the response by health professionals and the distortions and gaps in their knowledge and attitudes about this topic. This is not only a historical legacy, but in our contemporary world many of the issues faced in Western countries relating to IPA are similar.

In Chapter 2 Kelsey Hegarty gives more background to the succeeding chapters by addressing the question 'What is intimate partner abuse?' Inconsistent definitions of IPA in research and practice have resulted in varying estimates of its prevalence. She considers issues such as what relations should be termed 'domestic' and how violence in domestic life should be defined, and then discusses how the various definitions on which measures of IPA are based influence studies of prevalence rates throughout the world. Methodological issues in IPA research are discussed, including various theories of causation of IPA that influence researchers and practitioners in their methodologies and practice.

SECTION 2: IMPACT, EDUCATION, IDENTIFICATION, AND INTERVENTION

Section 2 is designed to inform health professionals on practical, educational, and legal aspects of IPA. It includes descriptions of the impact of IPA and how to intervene with those who experience it directly and indirectly. New approaches to education of health professionals and legal issues relevant to the topic of IPA are discussed. The basic principles of education of all health professionals and management of victims of IPA are similar, therefore the chapters are written in such a way as to be useful for a wide range of health disciplines. Each chapter refers to research evidence, and conclusions or recommendations make explicit reference to the nature of the evidence supporting them.

IPA is a significant risk factor for a wide range of physical and mental health problems. The impact of IPA is discussed in Chapter 3 by Jacquelyn Campbell and her colleagues. They present the clinical signs of IPA and the mechanisms explaining their presentation in various health care settings, as supported by both research and extensive clinical practice with women affected.

In addition to the need for acquiring new knowledge and skills, health professionals are faced with the task of confronting the feelings and social beliefs that shape their responses to those who experience IPA. Chapter 4 outlines new models for incorporating public health and advocacy-based principles into the education of heath professionals, working in partnership with community groups. Furthermore, it explores changes in the health care system itself.

The barriers to identification in health care settings, which include both the barriers to disclosure by women and inquiry by health professionals, are outlined in Chapter 5. Kelsey Hegarty and colleagues discuss the international debates around screening in health care settings. Evidence-based recommendations for health professionals about who they should be asking and how they should inquire are examined.

At present there is limited evidence about what works in different health care settings for women who have experienced IPA. In Chapter 6 Gene Feder and colleagues outline the research that has been conducted in the areas of advocacy and psychological interventions. Good practice in health care settings is embedded into a wider community response to IPA. The authors explore the limitations of the research base for guidelines to assist women who experience IPA and highlight priorities for future research.

In Chapter 7 Heather McCosker-Howard and Anne Woods discuss the impact of IPA on child-

bearing women, which encompasses maternal, fetal, and neonatal outcomes. Current approaches to the identification of women experiencing long- and short-term health sequelae from IPA are critically analysed from the perspective of the women and maternity health service providers. To encourage a coordinated response between current research knowledge and maternity health care, suggestions for evidence-based clinical practice, teaching, and directions for research are provided.

In the past decade, a growing number of empirical research studies have demonstrated that exposure to IPA has negative effects on children's social, emotional, and cognitive development, as well as their physical and mental health. In Chapter 8 Jennifer Smith summarizes research findings about the relationship between exposure to IPA and children's psychosocial adjustment. It is acknowledged that the research into clinical responses is in its infancy, and a brief overview of therapeutic interventions and techniques, and their effectiveness, is given.

Angela Taft and Judy Shakespeare provide an overview of the complexities in providing health care to men who abuse their partners and/or children, an area in which there is little research evidence at present. Chapter 9 provides an international perspective on the challenges of caring for the whole family in the context of abuse and addresses the intricacies and dilemmas for health care providers. Other challenges face clinicians: both men who abuse and women who are abused may also abuse their children; and older children, especially sons, can harm non-abusing parents. The authors outline presenting symptoms and current consensus about good management, including safety, confidentiality, and coordination issues when professionals are working with individuals, couples, or other family members. Attention is given to high-risk groups such as women and children in refuges, and women with disabilities. The issue of confidentiality versus responsibility to children at risk of harm is discussed.

In Chapter 10 Jocelynne Scutt provides useful information for health professionals on legal issues associated with IPA. She pursues the theme of women speaking to professionals, including police, the judiciary and health professionals, and not being heard. Her point is illustrated with a remarkable case study in Australia. Links between law and custom, the difference between civil and criminal law as it relates to IPA, information about protection orders for victims, government initiatives, and the importance of reports by health professionals and their evidence in court are important legal issues that are discussed. The advantages and disadvantages of the controversial issue of mandatory reporting are outlined.

SECTION 3: CULTURAL DIVERSITY AND INTIMATE PARTNER ABUSE

In Section 3 issues of cultural diversity and IPA in different ethnic groups are explored, as well as IPA in Indigenous peoples and people in same-sex relationships.

In Chapter 11 Michael Rodriguez and George Saba provide a background for the subsequent chapters with a discussion of cultural competence, a set of skills, behaviours, attitudes, and policies that can work effectively in a cross-cultural setting. This is particularly important because of the sensitivity needed to build bridges between those who experience IPA and health professionals who frequently have a different set of values and beliefs about the context and results of abuse. The chapter includes strategies to improve quality of care.

Judy Atkinson's Chapter 12 gives an international perspective on IPA and Indigenous people. The Indigenous family has to cope with the dominant societal and cultural constructions in the majority community. Some of these social and cultural practices promote individual, family, and community abusive behaviours, and dysfunction in minority communities. Within Indigenous families such behaviours must be seen in the context of a dominant society that has exerted power over, and used violence against them. Colonization has created situations where Indigenous women and children are particularly vulnerable. This chapter considers the documented extent of violence within the Australian Aboriginal context; the effects of violence on both victims and their families; actions of violence experienced as trauma; and the articulated need for 'healing' in the lives of those involved. Similarities and differences in principle and outcome for other colonized Indigenous peoples, such as those in the USA, Canada, and Aotearoa/New Zealand, are discussed.

IPA in same-sex relationships is poorly studied and not well understood in research or policy terms. The published research is clouded by small sample sizes, venue-based and snowball sampling methods, and theoretical challenges. In Chapter 13 Michael Relf and Nancy Glass provide an incisive critique of the existing literature, highlighting the prevalence of same-sex IPA, antecedents and outcomes, and barriers to identifying and treating the perpetrator and the victim. They conclude with recommendations for clinical training, including culturally competent assessment, and practice, policy, and research.

The final chapter makes recommendations based on the discussion of complex issues in this book, and outlines future directions in research and training for health professionals.

We hope you find this book useful for understanding IPA in the context of health and health services, examining your own practice, and supporting improved systems of care in your organization.

We wish to thank all the contributors, who have been very patient as we have returned draft after draft of their chapters. Also we thank our partners for their encouragement: John Roberts (Gwenneth's husband), Bill Harley (Kelsey's husband), and Sarah Mott (Gene's wife). We especially thank John Roberts for proof-reading the chapters. We acknowledge Catherine Jackson from Elsevier, who was always prompt to come to our assistance when problems occurred. Thank you to the Foreword writers, Beverley Raphael and Iona Heath, for their gracious assistance. Finally, we want to acknowledge the abused women throughout the world who have been our inspiration, many of whom pass through the health systems we have written about in this book. It is our hope that health professionals will be better informed about IPA and will be able to assist in a sensitive manner those women experiencing abuse whom they meet in the course of their practice.

REFERENCE

1. World Report on Violence and Health. Geneva: WHO; 2002. Available from: http://www.who.int/health_topics/violence/en/

SECTION 1

History and background issues

Chapter 1

The history of intimate partner abuse and health professionals: what have we inherited?

Gwenneth Roberts

Wife abuse takes place in the majority of societies . . . (and) has been condoned throughout most of history. Historically the tradition of accepting wife assault has been longer than the tradition of deploring it.[1]

INTRODUCTION

Historians who have addressed the topic of intimate partner abuse (IPA) agree that the most striking historical feature of the problem has been the intermittent nature of public concern about it.[2] It is difficult to find any written historical period in which there were no rules governing wife-beating and 'specifying the conditions under which a wife was deserving of a good clout'.[3] The lack of public discussion is the leading indicator for the necessity of a historical approach to understanding the way society and the health and legal professions have responded to IPA.

In the first part of this chapter the social, legal, and political factors associated with the occurrence of wife beating in nineteenth-century England and USA will be addressed. The rise of feminism in Western countries, and the response of health professionals to IPA will be explored. A discussion of the phenomenon of hysteria follows, and an examination of the literature investigates links between hysteria and physicians' attitudes to IPA. Research papers in the late twentieth century reveal the legacy of attitudes derived from psychoanalytic theories of the nineteenth century, attitudes which have influenced all health disciplines. Tensions between the battered women's movement and health professionals, and some shifts in the study of psychological trauma, will be explored. Finally, a description of how the nursing profession has responded to IPA will be described.

HISTORICAL BACKGROUND TO IPA

Allen, a feminist historian, described domestic violence as a 'practice without history'.[4] She considered that crimes such as woman-battering were a function of the secrets of sex and sexuality. Such crimes connected with relations between men and women could illuminate the generally secret characteristics of their negotiations. Sexuality was perhaps the most secret aspect of such negotiations and this secrecy could be identified as an obstacle to its historical investigation.

Pahl argues that one aspect of family life that was conducive to the occurrence of violence in the family, and has received little attention, was the dichotomy between public and private life.[5] The differentiation of public from private life could be seen running through political thought from the ancient Greeks to the present day. Thus a crime of violence committed in the home was seen as a different (lesser) sort of crime to violence against a stranger in a public place. The right to domestic privacy was more easily invoked and defended by some members of society than by others. In the context of wife abuse the privacy of the perpetrator may be respected at the expense of the well-being of the victim. Pahl saw this differential right to privacy as an important explanation of the 'invisibility' of wife abuse in most societies and in most periods of history. However, exceptions to invisibility are often found when feminist historical research is conducted. For instance, Dobash and Dobash[6] document concern about beaten women among the wives of the Roman senators. It may be that there is less invisibility in the historical record and more blindness to this issue among those who usually examine historical records.

Although IPA is an ancient problem particular emphases have been created in the public discussion by the lack of a history.[7] Two examples illustrate these emphases. One was the tendency of the nineteenth-century media to cover only the cruellest cases, creating the impression that these were typical. The problem gained attention through the most sensational cases, while most of the cases were ambiguous, not life-threatening, more often crimes of neglect than of assault. Another example was that many of the twentieth-century diagnoses of the causes of IPA, such as the increasing permissiveness of family life, assumed that the problem was unprecedented. The ebb-and-flow pattern of concern about family violence over the last century suggests that its incidence has not changed as much as its visibility, even in the absence of comparable and robust data.

Central to an understanding of the occurrence of IPA in any society is an examination of familial and household relations. One of the most fundamental aspects of these relations is how they change over time. Dolan focused on the discontinuity of representations of domestic crime.[8] For example, in the late sixteenth and seventeenth centuries, the murderous perpetrators who were the subjects of pamphlets dealing with domestic homicide were overwhelmingly wives and sometimes servants, although wives and servants actually were far more likely to be the victims of violence at the hands of male heads of households. This discrepancy is attributed to a cultural anxiety about murderous wives. In the late seventeenth century the murderous husband replaced the wife as the perpetrator of domestic murder in pamphlet literature. Murderous husbands were depicted as excessively violent or abusive, and portrayed as aberrations from the norm. Non-lethal violence and abuse were characterized as an acceptable part of male authority over women within the household. These attitudes were sanctioned by religious, political, and philosophical thinkers in the Western tradition and carried over to the nineteenth century.[3]

In a study of crimes of violence between working-class men and women in London, 1840–75, Tomes examined two types of violence – assaults by husbands on their wives, and assaults by men on women outside their family.[9] She found that women were the victims of aggravated assaults more often than men, and that wife-beating was common, accounting for about half of the cases. An examination of community responses and standards found that wife-beating was more readily tolerated than other forms of violence against women. Patterns of expectations held by men and women shaped their relationships. Male prerogative was based on financial support of his family, and violence erupted over money, drink, and authority. These and other characteristics of violent relationships such as provocation by the woman were considered causes of domestic violence, and have lingered to the present time.

Marriage in the second half of the nineteenth century, and especially middle-class marriage, was subjected increasingly to unprecedented public scrutiny and regulation. Demands for regulation came from a wide ideological spectrum, ranging from feminists to conservative moralists. The attitudes of some middle-class magistrates and judges who sentenced the perpetrators of violence changed. Increasingly, they viewed the physical abuse of women as 'barbaric', and called wife-beaters 'brutes' and 'tyrants'.[9]

Their viewpoints influenced changes in legislation; between 1840 and 1882, the maximum sentence for assaults on women was increased. In 1882, the Wife Beaters Act gave police magistrates the power to have offenders flogged and exposed on a public pillory.[9] Whilst this curtailed the most flagrant forms of abuse it left the usual patterns of patriarchal control unfettered and merely set the boundaries of what was considered 'normal'.[10] Judges still clung to the dictates of Common Law, and were influenced by ideas that criminal justice intervention would disrupt the domestic order.[11]

At the same time, these views were challenged by women campaigners in the community such as Frances Power Cobbe in England and Lucy Stone in the USA, who took up the cause of abused women in the nineteenth century. An earlier period of reform had taken place in American history. From 1640 to 1680, the Puritans of colonial Massachusetts enacted the first laws anywhere in the world against wife-beating and 'unnatural severity' to children. The second era of reform in American history occurred at the same time as the issue was being addressed in England (from 1874 to about 1890).[12] This took the form of societies for the prevention of cruelty to children, and smaller efforts were initiated on behalf of battered women and victims of incest.

Cobbe was concerned about the status of women in general, but particularly the plight of working-class wives. In a seminal article, 'Wife-Torture in England', which appeared in the April issue of *Contemporary Review* in 1878 she documented the horrors for these women.[13] However, the abuses she described were not confined solely to the lower classes. She asserted that many individuals of the upper class were more discreet in their abuse, making sure to direct their blows and kicks to those parts of the female anatomy that were not so obvious, such as the abdomen. Cobbe showed remarkable insights into IPA, and her language and understanding of the issue are still relevant to today's society. She was opposed to the flogging of a perpetrator, even though she called him a Beating Animal. Cobbe's campaign for improvement in civil law led to the passing of the Matrimonial Causes Act of 1878. This law made provision for women to obtain legal separation from violent husbands, and entitled them to maintenance and separation allowances and custody of their children.[13]

PSYCHIATRY AND IPA

Far removed from the feminist and the legal spheres were the emerging disciplines of psychiatry, psychoanalysis, and criminology in the late nineteenth and early twentieth centuries. In exploring their response to the topic of IPA it is important to contextualize it within the societal response to the issue because, as Mugford says, 'practitioners assume the broader community values [about domestic violence]'.[14] While this is true, other internal professional factors influenced the attitudes of health professionals to domestic violence in the nineteenth century.

A factor to be considered is the political context of the rise of contemporary psychiatry in the nineteenth century and its progression from Darwinian psychiatry to psychoanalysis. In the early part of the century the emerging discipline of psychiatry in Europe, with its enlightened-humanitarian scientific ethos clashed with proponents of a monarchy who supported the brutally punitive fanaticism of religion.[15] It is within this political context that the increase in the diagnosis of hysteria took place in Europe and America, an era that some have called 'the golden age of hysteria'.[16]

The psychiatric literature reveals the 'hiddenness' of IPA, and a detective exercise involves 'reading between the lines'. If IPA, or the equivalent terminology of the nineteenth century, such as 'wife-beating', was acknowledged, it was often embedded in a long list of other causative factors of a particular disease. Causes of hysteria included: 'impossibly stringent sexual and psychological demands placed upon women'[17] and 'traumatic domestic events such as physical maltreatment of the wife'.[18] These factors readily translate into characteristics of IPA as currently defined but there is little evidence that the health professionals addressed these particular problems. In the light of current evidence of the effects of domestic violence on women's mental health, it is very likely that women who had experienced IPA, as it is now defined, would have been presenting to nineteenth-century clinicians.[19,20] Symptoms reported by these women, such as headaches and pelvic pain, were diagnosed as hysteria. We now know that the diagnosis of somatization may be given to abused women. Recent research has noted the association between IPA and recurring central nervous system symptoms, including fainting and seizures, typical symptoms of hysteria.[21] The diagnosis of hysteria continued into the twentieth century.

Physicians whose works were influential in their time, and have only recently been acknowledged by historians, include Carter in England (1828–1918) and Briquet in France (1796–1881). Carter rejected the doctrine of a constitutional disposition to nervous disease, and refuted genital, visceral, and neurological causes of hysteria.[22] He replaced these with negative emotional experiences combined with an impressionable temperament, but argued that it was specifically the repression of strong feelings that produced hysteria. Carter acknowledged the social circumstances surrounding hysteria, and in comparing the emotional structure of men and women, he stated, 'the woman is more often under the necessity of endeavouring to conceal her feelings'.[23] It is highly unlikely that in this atmosphere women would reveal their experiences, or feelings about IPA, to the physician. Contemporary research has shown that the reasons why women do not disclose include guilt, shame, and embarrassment.[6,24] Given the role of the nineteenth-century woman as moral guardian of the family, these are feelings that she would be reluctant to reveal.

The traditions of English psychiatry during the nineteenth century were based on its belief that its therapeutic authority depended on domination over the patient's language. Carter told his colleagues, 'If a patient . . . interrupts the speaker, she must be told to keep silence and to listen; and must be told, moreover . . . in such a manner as to convey the speaker's full conviction that the command will be immediately obeyed'.[25] Insights into Carter's doctor–patient relationship are revealed in what is called 'medical moralizing'.[26] In describing the treatment of tertiary hysterical attacks that he considered initiated voluntarily by the patient, Carter presented a programme that was paternalistic in the extreme. He recommended that the physician would exercise 'complete control' over the patient. Again, it is unlikely that the woman would reveal IPA under these restraints.

The final development in the history of hysteria occurred in the late nineteenth century with a paradigm shift from the gynaecological, demonological, and neurological models of the past to a psychological theory. The most significant of these theories was Freudian psychoanalysis, which in essence began as a theory of hysteria. Practising in Vienna, Freud (1856–1939) learned of the treatment of a patient with hysteria by his colleague Breuer in 1880–82, the case of 'Anna O'. She was able to trace her hysterical symptoms back to specific emotionally disturbing events in her past, and in the course of remembering the traumatic scene she was able to bring the events into consciousness. This in turn caused the symptoms to disappear, a procedure the patient called 'the talking cure'. Freud adopted Breuer's method, naming it 'the cathartic method'.[27]

In Freud's paper entitled 'The aetiology of hysteria' (1896), he reported 18 cases of hysteria in adult patients. He postulated that 'at the bottom of every case of hysteria there are one or more occurrences of premature sexual experience, occurrences which belong to the earliest years of childhood'.[28] He conjectured that the repressed pathogenic material consisted of unconscious memories of childhood sexual traumas, experiences that could be reproduced by analytic work although whole decades have intervened. Freud considered that 'our children are far oftener exposed to sexual aggressions than we should suppose, judging by the scanty precautions taken by parents in this matter'.[29] Freud stated that the aetiological role of infantile sexual experiences was not confined to hysteria, but held good equally for other psychiatric disorders.[30] The recognition of child sexual abuse in women's lives is important because recent research has revealed that child sexual abuse is a risk factor for being abused in an adult intimate relationship.[31,32] The World Health Organization 'Report on violence and health' (2002) stated 'nearly 1 in 4 women may experience sexual violence by an intimate partner in their lifetime. For many young women, sexual violence begins in childhood and adolescence. In some countries, up to one-third of adolescent girls report forced sexual initiation.'[33]

A century later Freud's paper still rivals contemporary clinical descriptions of the effects of childhood sexual abuse.[34] Freud's original model, known as Seduction Theory, was a post-traumatic paradigm that placed emphasis on external stressor events, and he understood the interrelatedness of what today are the four diagnostic categories of post-traumatic stress disorder (PTSD) in the *Diagnostic and statistical manual of mental disorders*, 4th edition.[35] However, Freud found himself professionally isolated, and Freud's correspondence reveals that he was increasingly troubled by the radical social implications of his hypothesis.[36] In 1897 his ideas shifted and he repudiated his theory of the origins of hysteria, suggesting that the actual memories of the patients were composed of sexual desires and fantasies retained in the unconscious for purposes of self-defence. Freud's later concept helped delay the elaboration and replication of his original work, namely the relation of sexual abuse and hysteria, for nearly 80 years.[37]

Feminist scholarship, which is the basis for the largest body of recent scholarship on hysteria, notes that the early years of psychoanalysis offered a considerable advance over the biological determinism and moralism of Darwinian psychiatry, and laid the groundwork for listening to women. Freud and Breuer presented a sympathetic view of hysterical women, in contrast to the portraits of hysterical women by English and French physicians of the period. In England the medical responses to psychoanalysis were stated in *The British Medical Journal* in 1908, 'This method of psychoanalysis is in most cases incorrect, in many hazardous, and in all dispensable.'[38] The militant voices of suffragists and feminists suggested that resistance to listening to women's complaints was widespread across a range of male-dominated institutions.[39]

By the 1930s, psychoanalytic theories greatly affected the way that wife-beating was understood by health professionals, and affected the treatment of victims and perpetrators of family violence by psychiatrists and social workers in the USA. Psychoanalytic ideas helped to liberate the modern world from Victorian morality, and the rhetoric of male brutishness and his helpless victim all but disappeared. It was replaced by images of the seductive daughter, the nagging wife, and the lying hysteric. These new ideas undercut the moral outrage against family violence generated in the Victorian era and, along with other factors such as the effect of World War I on the role of women in society, contributed to its decline as a social issue.[39]

In 1930, Helene Deutsch, a follower of Freud, expounded the theory of female masochism in women who were beaten or raped.[40] Deutsch's theory became the dominant psychoanalytic explanation for the victimization of women and changed the nature of the debate about why women remained in violent relationships. Whereas pre-Freudian psychiatrists believed that women remained with men who mistreated them because they were stupid or feebleminded, psychoanalytic theory suggested that women derived psychic and sexual gratification from being beaten and humiliated.

Deutsch's ideas had a large, direct influence on psychiatric practice. The first psychoanalytic articles on rape, which appeared in the 1940s, noted the victim's unconscious desire to be raped.[41] When interviewing women who had been physically or sexually abused, psychiatrists preferred to concentrate more on the dysfunction of a woman's family of origin rather than ask direct questions about the extent of the abuse. What was considered as male brutishness of the nineteenth century was now seen as the proof of female frigidity, and perpetrators of family violence were no longer held responsible for having committed illegal or immoral acts. The result was that, in exploring other areas that they believed caused psychological problems, psychiatrists failed to deal with real and environmental factors such as trauma, and thus minimized the seriousness of family violence. These ideas can be seen directly in two papers on IPA from the 1960s and early 1970s.[42,43]

THEORIES OF IPA

Prior to 1970, theories on family violence had focused on the idea that domestic violence was the product of mental illness or psychological disorder and there was as much, if not more, concern with the individual pathology of the victim as there was with the aggressor, in many circumstances.[44]

Men who battered were presented as mentally ill, neurotic, or disturbed; female victims were also regarded as neurotic or mentally ill. It was from this theoretical approach that the 'blaming the victim' attitude was derived, theories that were still prevalent in papers written by some psychiatrists in the 1960s and 1970s.[45]

Sociologists considered that the psychoanalytic model led to a failure to consider social organizational factors that caused family violence, and these attitudes have carried over to today. Hotaling commented: 'Hospitals and doctors have often avoided these problems [of family violence] entirely or looked at them from a narrowly medical angle. The mental health system has had a tendency to treat victims as though they were responsible for their own abuse.'[46] In 1974 the first study of IPA in the USA based on social–psychological analysis offered an explanation not based on the mental illness of offender or victim.[47] (See Chapter 2 for further discussion of theories of causation.)

RESEARCH INTO IPA

Before the 1970s there was little research interest within health and social science fields in IPA, although there was a burgeoning interest in child abuse by paediatric radiologists who observed the long bone fractures of children. Kempe's seminal article on child abuse appeared in the *Journal of the American Medical Association* in 1962.[48] No reliable statistics on the incidence of IPA were available in the 1960s and it was assumed that child abuse and other forms of family violence were rare occurrences. The first large community studies of IPA conducted in the USA in 1979 and 1985 used a measuring tool, the Conflict Tactics Scale, which became the gold standard for many subsequent studies.[49] Criticisms of this scale were that it ignored the cultural, situational, and motivational contexts within which IPA occurs. These will be discussed further in the context of definitional issues in Chapter 2. The findings of these studies suggested a symmetrical nature of IPA, where women were equally as violent as men. The battle over the 'battered husband syndrome' commenced with those who explained the asymmetry of spouse abuse where women were the primary victims.[50] It is now generally accepted that, although women can be violent in relationships with men, and violence is also found in same-sex partnerships, the overwhelming health burden of IPA is borne by women at the hands of men.[33]

IPA AND HEALTH PROFESSIONALS IN THE TWENTIETH CENTURY

There was virtually no public discussion about wife-beating from the end of the nineteenth century until the mid-1970s. The second wave of feminism contributed to placing the issue of domestic violence on the public agenda. With the rise of the battered women's movement and the opening of women's shelters in the Western world, the women's movement challenged the police, social agencies, health professionals, and governments to respond adequately to the problem.[10] Research in clinical settings such as emergency departments, antenatal clinics, and psychiatric institutions revealed the high rates of survivors of IPA in those places.[51-53]

Subsequently, IPA has been recognized in Australia as a public health issue by bodies such as the Australian Medical Association[54] and the Public Health Association of Australia.[55] In an address to the Pan American Health Organization in 1989, the Surgeon General of the US Public Health Service stated that,

> Female abuse has been reported from almost every culture; it crosses all ethnic groups, races, religions and national boundaries . . . For whatever reasons, there has been a reluctance here and throughout the world to deal effectively with the global problem of violence against females. This has had the effect of trivializing a major problem of our times . . . It certainly is a public health problem of major proportions.[56]

Gradually clinical expertise was brought to bear on IPA, but not without depoliticizing it and psychologizing abuse in the process.[12] Arising out of the mental health professions, more particularly in the USA, and to a lesser degree in the UK and Australia, was a diagnostic approach to IPA. It was hypothesized that early social influences on women facilitated a psychological condition called 'learned helplessness', and that battered women were basically passive and submissive in response to abuse.[57] This theory was countered by researchers who demonstrated that battered women are help-seekers who persistently search for resources and support services, and that these same sources may not provide sufficient aid.[58] The 'battered woman syndrome' was a distinct social–psychological category that identified women experiencing persistent violence as having unique personality disorders. These concepts were widely accepted, and were commonly used in court cases, particularly as a defence for women who killed their husbands. Tensions arose with those in the women's movement who saw the diagnostic concepts as the antithesis of the visions of activists who sought social change. They claimed that the focus of therapy was interpersonal relationships and not the wider social, cultural, and political contexts of social problems that were the focus of the battered women's movement.[10]

Psychological trauma and IPA

A shift has taken place in the study of psychological trauma. Harvey presented a model that utilized an ecological view of psychological trauma and trauma recovery.[59] She proposed that individual differences in post-traumatic response and recovery are the result of complex interactions among person, event, and environmental factors. In attending to the social, cultural, and political context of victimization and acknowledging that survivors of traumatic experiences may recover without benefit of clinical intervention, the model highlights the phenomenon of resiliency, and the relevance of community intervention efforts. These interventions need not be initiated in competition with clinical care alternatives. Rather, a full spectrum of clinical, community, and societal interventions is needed.

Others have contextualized the study of psychological trauma within a political movement. Herman stated that, 'Not until the women's liberation movement of the 1970's was it recognized that the most common post-traumatic disorders are those not of men in war but of women in civilian life.'[60] She considers that history teaches us that without the context of a political movement – and she includes the organized efforts of soldiers after the Vietnam war – it has never been possible to advance the study of psychological trauma, and this knowledge could disappear. Herman observes 'Only after 1980, when the efforts of combat veterans had legitimated the concept of post-traumatic stress disorder, did it become clear that the psychological syndrome seen in survivors of rape, domestic battery, and incest was essentially the same as the syndrome seen in survivors of war.'[61] Now recent research is suggesting that although PTSD in women has similar elements to that experienced by males, gender differences are also important, perhaps because of the nature of the trauma usually experienced.[62]

Nursing and IPA

In 1984, Campbell and Humphreys published a ground-breaking text on the subject, *Nursing care of victims of family violence*.[63] The purpose of the book was to integrate nursing practice in family violence with existing theory and research. The authors identified that nursing had limited knowledge in this area, with other disciplines such as law and social work conducting most of the analysis and study. A discrepancy existed between the potential magnitude of the role of nursing in the care of violent families and the amount of nursing knowledge and research available, and increasing the latter was a consistent theme in the authors' book. They considered that, for nurses, awareness of the problem of family violence was not enough, and extended their role to that of victim advocates. From the time of Florence Nightingale, the professional nurse has been concerned with the individual, the family, and the community. Nurses were in an ideal position to take action to decrease the likelihood of family violence and mitigate against its effects because of their sheer numbers, predominantly female gender, variety of practice locations, and, in particular, the nature of their practice. Doctors had become aware of family violence, but they were criticized for the emphasis on physical symptomatology to alert them to its presence. Campbell and Humphreys stated 'The medical model generally leads to assumptions of pathology in victims as well as perpetrators, and treatment recommendations are usually in terms of psychiatric care. A nursing perspective would appropriately emphasize the healthy aspects of the families experiencing violence, an approach well supported by actual research on victims'.[64]

Nursing research has generally grown out of clinical concerns rather than a deductive theoretical testing approach. Nurse researchers have usually made suggestions for clinical interventions in their research reports. This reflects nurses' clinical background with battered women and their links with the women's shelter movement. Thus, nursing research has been congruent with the calls for a social research agenda, which has been proposed by other researchers with a feminist theoretical basis.[65] Nursing research in the USA has emphasized qualitative and phenomenological methods rather than quantitative research. This research has made the contrast with psychology, sociology, victimology, and women's studies that were more concerned with documenting emotional effects, and sociological and psychological factors. Nurse researchers have added both physical injury and physical responses to the emotional and behavioural reactions usually studied.[66] As a group of professionals who are likely to have a proportion of their members who have experienced IPA, nurses are in a unique position to address the problems of domestic violence as they relate to women's health.

The Nursing Network on Violence against Women International, which commenced in the USA in the early 1980s, exists as a loose coalition of nurses and other concerned advocates and health professionals. One of the main activities of this organization has been an ongoing collection of protocols and training manuals prepared by nurses for the care of battered women in health care settings.[67,68] Thus the nursing profession has joined other health professions in attempting to address the problems of IPA.

SUMMARY

In this brief chapter the invisibility of IPA throughout history as an issue on the public agenda and for health professionals has been established. The legacy that health professionals have inherited has been described from numerous sources: Greek political thought, nineteenth-century societal views of household and familial relations, feminist campaigners, psychoanalytic theory, the phenomenon of hysteria, sociologists, the diagnosis of 'battered woman syndrome', shifts in the study of psychological trauma, and the nursing profession. Although IPA has taken its place within the last thirty years on the public agenda, and has been recognized as a public health issue, there remain numerous aspects of this topic that still need to be addressed, such as education of health professionals; screening, identification, and intervention with victims of IPA; the impact of IPA on children and whole families; cross-cultural issues; and medico-legal issues such as mandatory reporting of abuse. The complexity of these aspects will be discussed in succeeding chapters. This book will endeavour to point the way forward for health professionals as they address the issue of IPA.

REFERENCES

1. Pahl J. Private violence and public policy: the needs of battered women and the response of the public services. London: Routledge; 1985:11.
2. May M. Violence in the family: an historical perspective. In: Martin J, ed. Violence and the family. Chichester: Wiley; 1978:135.
3. Bauer C, Ritt L. 'A Husband is a beating animal': Frances Power Cobbe confronts the wife-abuse problems in Victorian England. Int J Womens Stud 1983; 6(2):99–118.
4. Allen JA. Sex and secrets: crimes involving Australian women since 1880. Melbourne: Oxford University Press; 1990. *The central thesis of Allen's book 'Sex and secrets' was that crime historians' a priori confidence in the representativeness of crime trends and the significance of visible official actions was misplaced. She argued that the illicit practices that were not policed, or under-policed, or erratically policed, were at least as historically significant as those criminalities which were most policed. Sex has been of central cultural significance in modern Australian history and it is a key dimension of historical subjects. Historical evidence can reveal an investment of authorities and institutions in the secrets and secrecy of sex. They have been reluctant to intervene or publicize even when one party to the secret (such as a victim of rape) demanded redress through the criminal justice system.*

5. Pahl J. Private violence and public policy: the needs of battered women and the response of the public services. London: Routledge; 1985.

6. Dobash RE, Dobash RP. Violence against wives. London: Open Books; 1979.

7. Gordon L. Heroes of their own lives: the politics and history of family violence, Boston 1880–1960. New York: Viking Penguin; 1988. *Gordon's historical research consisted of a case-study of how the Boston-area social work agencies approached family violence problems, from 1880 to 1960. She argued that, although the data in this book came exclusively from the Boston metropolitan area, which had certain demographic and social peculiarities, there was reason to consider the findings of this study typical of the urban United States. The largest environmental factors affecting family violence (e.g. poverty, unemployment, illness, alcoholism) were common to many areas. Moreover, the 'discovery' of this social problem occurred simultaneously throughout the United States and in much of Europe, in the course of a single decade, suggesting similar patterns.*

8. Dolan F. Dangerous familiars: representations of domestic crime in England, 1550–1700. London: Cornell University Press; 1994. *Dolan attempts to chart how representations of domestic violence, in the form of pamphlets, ballads, plays, and trial transcripts, shaped and were shaped by early modern cultural practices, with chapters on spousal murder, petty treason by wives and servants, infanticide, and witchcraft.*

9. Tomes N. A 'Torrent of abuse': Crimes of violence between working-class men and women in London, 1840–1875. J Soc Hist 1978; 11:328–345. *This study is based on a sample of 100 cases of violence between men and women taken from both the sessions papers of the Central Criminal Court of London and the trial accounts published daily in the London Times. Tomes acknowledges that statistics for her study of records in the London police courts were not consistent, and that there remains a 'dark figure', including assaults that were never reported to the police.*

10. Dobash RE, Dobash RP. Women, violence and social change. London: Routledge; 1992.

11. Cox E. The principles of punishment. London: Law Times Office; 1877.

12. Pleck E. Domestic tyranny: the making of social policy against family violence from colonial times to the present. New York: Oxford University Press; 1987.

13. Cobbe Frances Power. Wife-torture in England. Contemporary Review 1878; 32:56–87.

14. Mugford J. Domestic violence. Canberra: National Committee on Violence; 1989.

15. Goldstein J. Hysteria diagnosis and the politics of anticlericalism in late nineteenth century France. J Mod Hist 1984; 54:209–239.

16. Micale MS. Hysteria and its historiography: the future perspective. Hist Psychiatry [Great Britain] 1990; 1(1):39.

17. Carter RB. On the pathology and treatment of hysteria. London: John Churchill; 1853:33.

18. Mai FM. Pierre Briquet: nineteenth century savant with twentieth century ideas. Can J Psychiatry 1981; 28(1):57–63.

19. Golding JM. Intimate partner violence as a risk factor for mental disorders: a meta-analysis. J Fam Violence 1999; 14:99–132.

20. Roberts GL, Lawrence JM, Williams GM, et al. The impact of domestic violence on women's mental health. Aust N Z J Public Health 1998; 22(7):56–61.

21. Campbell JC. Health consequences of intimate partner violence. Lancet 2002; 359:1331–1336.

22. Carter RB. On the pathology and treatment of hysteria. London: John Churchill; 1853.

23. Veith I. Hysteria: the history of disease. Chicago: University of Chicago Press; 1970:202.

24. Roberts GL. Domestic violence victims in the Emergency Department. Doctoral dissertation (unpublished), University of Queensland, Australia; 1995.

25. Carter RB. On the pathology and treatment of hysteria. London: John Churchill; 1853:43.

26. Micale MS. Hysteria and its historiography: a review of past and present writings. Hist Sci 1989; 27(1):223–261.

27. Freud S. The aetiology of hysteria. In: Sutherland JS, ed. Collected Papers, Vol. 1. London: Hogarth Press; 1957:185.

28. Ibid. 193.

29. Ibid. 203.

30. Ibid. 217.

31. Beitchman JH, Zucker KJ, Hood JE, et al. A review of the long-term effects of child sexual abuse. Child Abuse Neglect 1992; 16:101–118.

32. Fleming J, Mullen PE, Sibthorpe B, et al. The long-term impact of childhood sexual abuse in Australian women. Child Abuse Neglect 1999; 23:145–159.

33. World Report on Violence and Health. Geneva: WHO; 2002. Available from: http://www.who.int/health_topics/violence/en/

34. Herman JL. Trauma and recovery. London: Basic Books; 1992:13.

35. Wilson J. The historical evolution of PTSD diagnostic criteria: from Freud to DSM-IV. J Trauma Stress 1994; 7(4):681–698.

36. Bonaparte M, Freud A, Kris E, eds. The origins of psychoanalysis: letters to Wilhelm Fliess, drafts and notes, 1887–1902; by Sigmund Freud. New York: Basic Books; 1954, 215–216.

37. Pynoos RS. Post-traumatic symptoms in incest victims. In: Eth S, Pynoos RS, eds. Post-traumatic stress disorders in children. Washington, DC: American Psychiatric Press; 1985.

38. Weeks J. Sex, politics and society. London: Longman; 1981:142.

39. Showalter E. The female malady: women, madness and English culture 1830–1980. New York: Pantheon Books; 1985:162.

40. Deutsch H. The significance of masochism in the mental life of women. Int J Psychoanal 1930; 5(11):48–60.

41. Albin RS. Psychological studies of rape. Signs 1977; 3(2):427–429.

42. Snell JE, Rosenwald RJ, Robey A. The wife-beater's wife. Arch Gen Psychiatry 1964; 11:107–112.

43. O'Brien JE. Violence in divorce prone families. J Marriage Fam 1971; 33(4):692–698.

44. Schultz LG. The wife assaulter. J Soc Ther 1960; 6(2):103–111.

45. Scott PD. Battered wives. Br J Psychiatry 1974; 125:433–441.

46. Hotaling GT, Finkelhor D, Kirkpatrick JT, et al. Coping with family violence: research and policy perspectives. Newbury Park, CA: Sage; 1988:13.

47. Gelles RJ. The violent home. Updated edn. Newbury Park, CA: Sage; 1987.

48. Kempe CH, Silverman FN, Steele BF, et al. The battered-child syndrome. JAMA 1962; 181(1):105–112.

49. Straus MA. Measuring intra-family conflict and violence: The Conflict Tactics (CT) Scales. J Marriage Fam 1979; 41:75–88.

50. Steinmetz, SK. The battered husband syndrome. Victimology 1977–1978; 2:499–502.

51. Roberts GL, O'Toole BI, Raphael B, et al. Prevalence study of domestic violence victims in an emergency department. Ann Emerg Med 1996; 27(6):747–753.

52. Stark E, Flitcraft A, Zuckerman D, et al. Wife abuse in the medical setting: an introduction for health personnel. Rockville, MD: National Clearinghouse on Domestic Violence; 1981.

53. Webster J, Sweett S, Stolz TA. Domestic violence in pregnancy: a prevalence study. Med J Australia 1994; 161(8):466–470.

54. Doctor's role in domestic violence cases. Australian Medicine 1989; 1:373–374.

55. Domestic violence. In: Public Health Association of Australia – Policy Statements. Public Health Association of Australia; 1990:4.

56. Domestic violence: a guide for health care professionals. State of New Jersey: Department of Community Affairs; 1990.

57. Walker LE. The battered woman. New York: Harper and Row; 1979.

58. Gondolf EW, Fisher ER. Battered women as survivors: an alternative to treating learned helplessness. Lexington, MA: Lexington Books; 1988.

59. Harvey MR. An ecological view of psychological trauma and trauma recovery. J Trauma Stress 1996; 9(1):3–23.

60. Herman JL. Trauma and recovery. London: Basic Books; 1992:28.

61. Ibid. 32.

62. Woods SJ, Campbell JC. Posttraumatic stress in battered women: does the diagnosis fit? Issues Ment Health Nurs 1993; 14(2):173–186.

63. Campbell JC, Humphreys J, eds. Nursing care of victims of family violence. Reston, VA: Reston; 1984.

64. Ibid. 7.

65. Dobash RE, Dobash RP. Research as social action: the struggle for battered women. In: Yllo K, Bograd M, eds. Feminist perspectives on wife abuse. Newbury Park, CA: Sage; 1988:51.

66. Campbell JC. Health consequences of intimate partner violence. Lancet 2002; 359:1331–1336.

67. Helton AS. Protocol of care for the battered woman. Houston: Texas Women's University; 1986.

68. King MC, Perry M, Ryan J, et al. Reaching out to battered women: a training curriculum for nurses. Amherst, MA: NNVAW; 1987.

Chapter 2

What is intimate partner abuse and how common is it?

Kelsey Hegarty

At the time I felt that it was not really abuse but the longer I thought about it the more that I felt it was abuse. Emotional abuse is more severe than physical abuse as there is no outward marks or bruises. When this was realized by myself I got out. Living alone is far better than what was happening in the relationship.

CHAPTER CONTENTS

INTRODUCTION

The concept of domestic violence or intimate partner abuse (IPA) remains problematic, in both theoretical and practical terms, despite the attention it has been given by researchers, policy makers, clinicians, and activists. The growing volume of literature has not resolved debate about how these terms are defined. Inconsistent definitions in research and practice have contributed to the wide variation in estimates of its prevalence and associations with personal and social factors.[1] The unresolved issues include determining which relationships are domestic or intimate and agreement on definitions of violence and abuse. The chapter begins with these definitional issues and then briefly discusses theories of causation of intimate partner violence as background to the debate. It is also important to understand how definitions are operationalized by the measures used in research studies. How this has influenced the prevalence rates found throughout the developed world will be discussed, thus enabling practitioners to understand the variation in these rates from different studies. Selected examples of studies in community and clinical settings are then used to illustrate issues, drawing on reviews of studies where they exist.

WHAT IS IPA?

Domestic violence is sometimes used to refer to violence and abuse that occurs in any relationship within households in our communities, although it usually refers to partner abuse. Another term, 'family violence', refers to violence occurring between any family members. More recently, the Centers for Disease Control (CDC) and the World Health Organization (WHO) have recommended the more precise term 'intimate partner violence'.

Definition of intimate partner violence

- Physical and/or sexual violence (use of physical force) or threat of such violence; or psychological/emotional abuse and/or coercive tactics when there has been prior physical and/or sexual violence between persons who are spouses or non-marital partners (dating, boyfriend–girlfriend) or former spouses or non-marital partners (CDC).[2]
- Any behavior within an intimate relationship that causes physical, psychological, or sexual harm to those in the relationship; it includes: physical aggression, psychological abuse, forced intercourse and other forms of sexual coercion, various controlling behaviors (WHO).[3]

In some countries 'partner violence' has a legal meaning referring exclusively to heterosexual relationships where the couple have been or are cohabiting. Many feminists avoid the term 'domestic' or 'partner' and prefer 'wife assault' or 'battered women' to reflect the most common victims.[4-6] Partner abuse against women is likely to be a different form of domestic violence from elder abuse or sibling abuse because it converges with the broader patterns of discrimination against women in society.[5,7,8] The terms 'violence', 'abuse', and 'battering' are frequently used interchangeably, although such terms are often defined in different ways by researchers. For example, Straus[9] defined 'violence' as 'an act carried out with the intention, of, or perceived intention, of causing physical pain or injury to another person'. From a health perspective, IPA can be better understood as a chronic syndrome that is characterized not by the episodes of physical violence that punctuate the problem but by the emotional and psychological abuse that the perpetrator uses to maintain control over his partner. Furthermore, as most survivors of partner abuse report, the physical violence is the least damaging abuse they suffer: it is the relentless psychological abuse that cripples and isolates the woman.[10–12] Thus the term 'violence' is limiting for practical purposes and the term 'abuse' is preferable because it is inclusive of the varying actions that perpetrators use to control their partners.[13,14] Alexander[15] suggests a comprehensive definition of 'violence' that takes into account the varying types of abuse (emotional, physical, and sexual), severity and frequency of the abuse, and the intention and meaning of the abuse. The terms 'intimate partner violence' (IPV) and 'intimate partner abuse' (IPA) are used interchangeably throughout this chapter and the book.

Types of abuse

The Australian Public Health Association employs a broad definition that includes abuse of a physical, sexual, or emotional nature, with examples as outlined below:[16]

- Physical abuse causing pain and injury, denial of sleep, warmth, or nutrition, denial of needed medical care, sexual assault, violence to property or animals, disablement and murder;
- Verbal abuse in private or in public, designed to humiliate, degrade, demean, intimidate, subjugate, including the threat of physical violence;

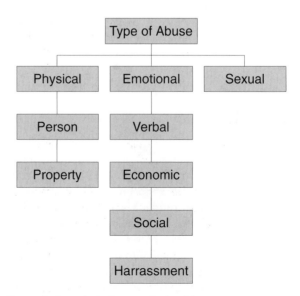

Figure 2.1   Types of abuse in intimate relationships.

- Economic abuse, including deprivation of basic necessities, seizure of income or assets, unreasonable denial of the means necessary for participation in social life; and
- Social abuse through isolation, control of all social activity, deprivation of liberty, or the deliberate creation of unreasonable dependence.

The CDC definition outlined earlier in this chapter only includes emotional abuse that is combined with physical or sexual violence, whilst the WHO definition includes psychological abuse by itself.

Severity and frequency of abuse

The definition and subsequent measurement of IPA are influenced by notions of acceptable and non-acceptable behaviour embedded in the norms and cultures of different societies. In addition, statistics on severity of physical violence tend to focus on physical injury requiring medical attention. As outlined previously, Straus[9] distinguished between minor and severe violence on the basis of the type of physical act and the likelihood of causing injury. Both of these methods are problematic because it is unknown whether injury as a consequence of physical violence correlates with survivors' own perceptions of the severity of the abuse they are experiencing. We learn nothing about the severity of emotional threats or the actual impact of physical acts on women's emotional states, for example.

Frequency interacts with severity because it may be that a frequent but more minor violent act (e.g. slapping) is equally damaging both in terms of physical injury and emotional harm to a victim compared to a more severe but once-only act (e.g. kicking). It is difficult to determine accurately how frequently physical violence needs to occur before it is classified as 'abuse' rather than as part of ordinary human conflict interaction. Much depends on the circumstances in which women find themselves, perceptions, norms, culture, and social relationships, all matters difficult to incorporate into an objective classification system. However, 'abuse' occurs where violence is embedded in coercive control of one human being over another and is not acceptable in any culture.

Meaning and intention of abuse

Significantly lacking in definitions and measurement of abuse has been the meaning and intention of such abuse. An exploration of intention could differentiate between isolated acts of physical violence, which are part of conflict between intimates, and intentionally coercive acts, which are part of a broader spectrum of behaviours that include physical, emotional, and sexual abuse. Dobash and Dobash[17] found intention to inflict harm or punish and control partners was a facet of men who frequently use violence against their partners. Episodes of once-only violence that are part of conflict in the relationship but are not embedded in other coercive tactics are thought not to be part of partner abuse by some researchers.[18–20] The next section explores which behaviours are classified as IPA by the general community.

Classification of domestic violence

There has been little systematic research into what constitutes IPV from a community viewpoint. An example from Australia highlights this issue, involving three studies commissioned by the federal Office of Status of Women. The first, completed in late 1987, was a survey of general community attitudes, and was repeated in 1995.[21] Another study in 1988 was an in-depth study of community and domestic violence professionals' attitudes.[22]

Using a checklist of possible behaviours that might constitute domestic violence, the 1987 survey showed that almost all respondents said that physical acts such as pushing, shoving, kicking, and choking should be classified as domestic violence. Domestic violence was taken to mean physical violence between partners usually perpetrated by the husband on the wife. The more recent survey (n = 2,004 adults) found that by 1995 there was a much broader definition of domestic violence. When asked about the main forms of domestic violence, 8 in 10 people mentioned physical violence but 6 in 10 also mentioned psychological abuse. Two-thirds of people classified denial of money as abuse in 1995 compared with one-quarter in 1987, and 80% of people classified verbal abuse as domestic violence in 1995, compared with about half in 1987. In all categories, women are more likely to be aware of psychological abuse than men are and attach a greater degree of seriousness to such abuse. Both men and women see men as much more frequent perpetrators.

In the 1988 study, victims, and professionals working with victims, mentioned physical abuse first when discussing what they considered domestic violence to be, but went on to discuss emotional (verbal abuse, social abuse, economic abuse) and sexual abuse.[22] As Mugford[23] points out, the above result shows that those who are well acquainted with the behaviour have no doubt that non-physical forms of abuse can be just as damaging as physical acts. In contrast, those in the general community are inclined to place less emphasis on non-physical behaviours. To understand the origin of these different views, it is instructive to overview the main theories of causation of IPV.

THEORIES OF CAUSATION

The abundance and variety of theories about the causes of IPA may reflect the likelihood of multiple causes or that there are several different patterns of abuse rather than a single entity of partner abuse against women. The origins of the various theories are still reflected in practice, research, and community attitudes. Early investigations in the 1960s focused on identification of personality traits that would cause men to attack their wives and women to accept the violence (see Chapter 1). Subsequent research in the 1970s developed various sociological, social–psychological, ecological, and multidimensional theories. More recently societal theories have arisen as part of the feminist movement. The three main frameworks for looking at domestic violence – the psychological, the sociological, and the feminist – are described below.

Psychological

Early psychological theory assumed that one or both partners possessed certain characteristics that made them prone to partner abuse. Initially IPV was felt to be a result of mental illness in both partners. This was discounted when it became obvious that domestic violence was highly prevalent in the community.[24] Subsequently, women were felt to be masochistic and men to have individual problems with loss of control. Critics of the individual psychopathology theories outline how studies of victims often confuse the symptoms resulting from the abusive behaviour (e.g. depression, anxiety) with the victim's own personality.[4] Another limitation of this approach has been the discovery that perpetrators do not have difficulty controlling their anger in any situations other than in the home, discounting hypotheses regarding poor impulse control.

Almost all current literature in this area is critical of the individual and psychoanalytical approach to causation of domestic violence because of its negative stance towards women.[25,26] The universal position adopted by current perspectives does not see women as the cause of the violence. Such a perspective has not stopped some health practitioners from 'blaming the victim'. Practitioners still frequently raise such questions as 'What did you do that made him hit you?' and 'Why do you stay with him?' in consultations with women experiencing abuse.[27,28]

Social learning theorists attribute violence in the home to a learnt behaviour from role modelling by parents who fought in their families of origin. There is some evidence to support this assertion.[29,30] Male perpetrators and female victims appear more likely to come from homes where their fathers beat their mothers.[31,32] The American Public Health Association reviewed the research, which indicates that while intergenerational transmission of violent intrafamilial relationships is not inevitable, children reared in violent homes are at an elevated risk of becoming abusers themselves in adulthood, thus perpetuating a cycle of violence.[33] However, a large number of perpetrators were not abused as children, nor came from violent homes.[34,35]

Sociological

Some sociological theorists do not specify IPA as distinct from other forms of family violence and draw on the conflict literature to view physical violence as one form of dispute between intimates.[36] At the core of this perspective is the view that social structures (e.g. work and family) have an effect on people that results in their violent behaviour. More recently, some sociologists have set out to identify risk factors and predictors of violence. These factors include age, sex, socioeconomic indicators, race, stress, and alcohol use.[37] In the late 1970s, alcohol, and stress from work, poverty, or unemployment were frequently cited as the underlying causes of the violence.[38] Evidence for this was usually from studies on victims and their associations with particular factors. Research thus far has been inconclusive about whether victims and their perpetrators are more likely to abuse alcohol than non-victims and their partners, and most importantly whether such a disproportionate risk preceded or followed the onset of abuse. A review of evidence for risk factors showed that violence in the family of origin of victim and perpetrator and unemployment of the perpetrator were the only variables that had sound evidence of an association.[28] Thus, with the exception of unemployment, none of the socioeconomic variables have been shown to be significant in predicting abuse by themselves. It is rather that the combination of environmental, social, and economic factors may contribute to IPV.

Feminist

By contrast, researchers and practitioners with a feminist perspective view partner abuse against women as a form of social control that emerges directly from the patriarchal structure and the ideology of the family.[5,7,39–41] To support this position there is historical evidence for the acceptance of wife-beating from biblical and medieval times (see Chapter 1).[42] Bograd[43] outlines that violence often occurs when women are failing to meet the traditional role of 'the good wife'. The least amount of abuse appears to occur in democratic or egalitarian households[44] and this is confirmed across several societies.[45]

A review of 29 studies[46] examined the predicted relation between wife assault and the maintenance of patriarchal ideology and found partial support for this theory. While violent males are more accepting of the use of violence against their wives, empirical evidence linking this violence to issues of traditional gender attitudes is limited. From a wider viewpoint, it has been argued that patriarchy promotes economic and legal conditions that maintain wife-beating.[7] Although feminist researchers view all domestic violence as a reflection of unequal power relationships, they have not rejected the relevance of social stresses, instead arguing that these are not a sufficient explanation.[34]

Which theory to adopt?

Which theory a practitioner or researcher adopts influences significantly their approach to interventions for partner abuse victims and also the methodologies applied in research. Yet no one theory fully explains the phenomenon of domestic violence. Unfortunately, a strong belief in only one explanatory framework has limited our understanding of IPA. Family Violence sociologists[37,47] saw the family as a site of conflict that reflects the broader societal conflict that exists between men and women. By contrast, Violence against Women researchers[7,48] view male to female aggression in relationships as coercive and that female to male aggression is usually in self-defence.[41,49–51] This contrast is most significantly demonstrated in our understanding of the victim. Family Violence researchers using surveys in the United States have revealed a gender equivalence of the violence that occurs between partners.[37,47] In contrast, Violence against Women researchers, using police reports, crime surveys, and qualitative methods, are convinced of a gender imbalance in violence, which occurs in partner relationships. Family Violence researchers have certainly demonstrated that there is equivalence in relationships with regard to particular violent acts, e.g. hitting with an object, but this is insufficient to constitute equivalence of partner abuse overall.

Current perspectives

To summarize, some researchers and practitioners do not view all violent behaviour between partners as IPV, depending on the context of the violent act. Whilst violent behaviour is never desirable, no great harm may accrue in instances where the partners regard and experience each other as equals and can give as good as they get back and where such instances are infrequent.[52] Lower levels of physical aggression (pushing, slapping, and shoving) which occur very frequently in couples in early marriage is not seen as abusive by either partner and is usually not in self-defence.[52] Other researchers and practitioners would classify all acts of violence within relationships as IPV.[47]

Many studies are not easily comparable because there is variation and insufficient standardization of criteria. Furthermore, researchers using different methodologies are often at cross-purposes when discussing partner abuse against women. Survey research using the Conflict Tactics Scale utilizes the physical abuse concepts outlined by Straus.[53–55] Other researchers utilizing interview methods describe a broader range of partner abuse.[25,48] These researchers and most practitioners see it as a complex pattern of behaviours that includes emotional, physical, and sexual abuse, not just simple physical acts of violence.[56,57] Partner abuse is seen as more likely to occur in a context of unequal power relationships within the family, where social attitudes support male authority over the family, and women's unequal access to economic security and domestic violence is a private concern rather than a public issue.[25] Assuming this to be the case, the question still remains why some individuals appear more prone to the negative influences of a patriarchal society than others do. In addition, sociologists employing national survey methodologies have found associations between domestic violence and age, marital status, and unemployment suggesting that characteristics in the social structure give rise to violence.[35,58]

Not all violent behaviour between partners may constitute partner abuse. Johnson[18] argues that there are two forms of violence against women. He suggests that some families suffer from occasional outbursts of violence during conflicts from either husbands or wives (common couple violence), and other families are terrorized by systematic male violence (patriarchal terrorism), while still other families may experience both. Similarly, Neidig,[19] in his discussion on physical abuse, outlines two types of violence, 'expressive' and 'instrumental', that occur in relationships. He proposes that an individual could be located at any point between these two extremes. Expressive violence occurs as a result of escalating conflict between partners, where it is easy to identify the precipitating event and both partners are involved in the escalation, although not equally. Instrumental violence is the deliberate use of violence as a tool to punish or control the behaviour of the partner. Furthermore, in the case of emotional abuse, conflicts in non-abusive relationships may be characterized at times by verbal aggression or withdrawal of affection on the part of either partner, but isolation from friends, family, and outside resources, and demands for subservience may be more characteristic of men who abuse.[50]

There may be several different patterns of violence and abuse in intimate relationships.[59] The first type of violence between partners might be infrequent, isolated minor physical acts (e.g. pushing and shoving) and minor emotional acts (e.g. withholding affection, saying spiteful things) that occur as part of conflicts amongst discordant partners or abused partners. Another type of violence is moderate to severe intermittent physical and/or sexual abuse combined with regular emotional abuse that occurs as part of coercive or control tactics mainly used by male partners against women. This is usually what practitioners describe when discussing the issue of partner abuse or domestic violence.[27] Furthermore, emotional abuse and physical abuse can occur by themselves and are likely to have different aetiologies and patterns to combined abuse.[60,61] The next section returns to the issues of definition and how those definitions are operationalized by the measures that are used in prevalence studies. This will enable an understanding of the variance in prevalences found in the different studies.

HOW IS IPV MEASURED?

Before looking at how common IPA is in health settings, it is important to discuss how it is measured. There are several instruments available for measuring partner abuse in the population (see Table 2.1). The Conflict Tactics Scale (CTS)[36] attempts to measure verbal and physical aggression and has been used in most research as the gold standard for domestic violence measurement.[62] Straus[47] operationalized 'abuse' in the CTS by identifying certain physical acts as being inherently 'abusive'. Thus any hitting of a partner is 'abuse', whilst only severely violent acts (kicking, beating up, choking, and threatening to use, or using a knife or gun) are 'wife-beating' or 'battering'. It has been criticized, however, for four main reasons.[24,42,63] First, it was developed to measure conflict tactics as opposed to coercive tactics. Second, the scale concentrates mainly on physical abuse, ignores sexual abuse, and has only limited items of verbal aggression.[24] Third, measurement error may also be common in survey studies utilizing the CTS because it does not elicit information about the intensity, context, consequences, or meaning of the action and most studies do not seek this information separately.[64] This lack of information on the consequences of the action means some items are classified as minor, e.g. slapping, which could in theory cause quite severe injury when perpetrated by a male. Furthermore, a respondent who indicates that they have slapped their partner twice is considered the same as one who indicates that they have been beaten up twice. Similarly, one qualitative study that conducted in-depth follow-up interviews following use of the CTS showed that respondents interpret the items positively even if the action is a mutually playful combat that is not harmful in any way to either partner.[65] The fourth problem is that the CTS is employed in summarized format to describe individual experiences of violence with no reference to duration or persistence or severity. Thus individuals can be labelled as victims because of one episode of 'tried to hit'. Gender equivalence of the perpetrators of violence is often the result of inclusion of these minor incidents even though qualitative data would suggest that self-defence is a common reason women hit their partners.[24,65] The CTS, however, does not measure a more comprehensive definition of IPA that incorporates emotional, physical, and sexual abuse.

The Revised Conflict Tactics Scale (CTS2) addresses some of the above issues but still has several major problems.[62] The refinement of the violence scales and the new injury scale should give some indication of the conse-

Table 2.1 Scales used frequently to measure IPA

Name (year)	Abuse types	No. of items	No. of respondents	Factors
Conflict Tactics Scale (1979)	Physical	8	2,143 undergraduate students	Violence
Index of Spouse Abuse (1981)	Physical Emotional	30	398 and 188 undergraduate female students	Physical Non-physical
Psychological Maltreatment of Women Inventory (1989)	Emotional	58	407 male abusers and 207 abused women	Domination/Isolation Emotional/Verbal
Abuse Behaviour Inventory (1992)	Physical Emotional	30	78 female partners of men in chemical dependency treatment	Psychological Physical
Severity Violence Against Women Scale (1992)	Physical Sexual	46	707 undergraduate students 200 community women	Symbolic violence Threats of violence: mild, moderate, severe Actual violence: mild, moderate, severe Sexual violence
Measure of Wife Abuse (1993)	Physical Sexual Emotional	60	165 abused women at shelters	Physical Verbal Psychological Sexual
Revised Contact Tactics Scale (1996)	Physical Sexual Emotional	39 Short-form 20	Undergraduate students	Physical assault Injury Sexual coercion Psychological aggression
Composite Abuse Scale (1999)	Physical Sexual Emotional	30	500 nurses and 1,896 general practice patients	Severe combined abuse Physical abuse Emotional abuse Harassment

quences of violent actions. However, the new psychological aggression items (e.g. 'shouted or yelled at my partner', 'accused partner of being a lousy lover', 'called my partner fat or ugly'), whilst extending the old verbal aggression scale, do not include any emotional abuse items, which are a prominent feature of partner abuse against women (e.g. social isolation and harassment). There is a new sexual coercion scale that once again has left out some sexual abuse acts against women (e.g. forced me to have sex with other partners). Straus[62] restates that the CTS is intended to be used in conjunction with other variables such as balance of power, feelings of fear, and intimidation. Unfortunately, however, the definition of partner abuse is often operationalized by researchers utilizing the CTS as one episode of minor violence and this is unlikely to change with the CTS2.

Three questionnaires – the Index of Spouse Abuse,[66] the Measure of Wife Abuse,[64] and the Abuse Behaviour Inventory[67] – attempt to measure the full range of forms of abuse but have only been validated on small samples. The Composite Abuse Scale (CAS) has four dimensions, which reflect women's experience of abuse: Severe Combined Abuse, Emotional Abuse, Physical Abuse, and Harassment. Three sample populations – a nurse ($n = 427$), general practice patient ($n = 1,836$), and emergency department patient ($n = 325$) – were used in the development and testing of the CAS.[68] The Severity of Violence Against Women Scales[69] only include acts which carry some amount of physical threat, but do include physical and emotional consequences of a range of severity of violent acts. Another scale, the Psychological Maltreatment of Women Inventory,[49] has been developed that focuses solely on emotional abuse. How these measures are used in prevalence studies in the community and clinical settings will be examined in the next section.

HOW COMMON IS IPA IN THE COMMUNITY?

There have been many debates in the literature and media about the extent of partner abuse against women. Prevalence studies are attempts to estimate the proportion of a population that has suffered partner abuse during adult life or in a specified time period. This is in contrast to incidence studies, which estimate the number of new cases occurring in a given time period. It is more common for studies to report prevalence than incidence. In the last decade, the number of prevalence studies in this area has increased dramatically although there has been a marked variation in the rates reported by different researchers.

In USA studies, it has been found that partner abuse may involve from 5% to 20% of the population of the USA, depending on the criteria used for the definition of partner abuse.[40] Definitions range from physical abuse in current relationships to inclusion of emotional and sexual abuse in past relationships. A study examined a representative sample of domestic violence investigations and found that only 16% even described the criteria used to define the abused sample.[70] The recent WHO Violence Against Women report[2] revealed that in 48 population-based surveys around the world, 10–69% of women had been physically assaulted by their partners at some stage in their lives. Heise[71] reviewed data available from random community samples in non-English-speaking countries and found rates of physical abuse (with sample sizes of around 1000) as high as 30–50% for urban and rural women in countries such as Barbados, Kenya, India, Malaysia, Colombia, Costa Rica, Guatemala, Mexico, and Chile. There was no description of the definition of wife abuse used but the sample size and methodology were outlined for each study. In Australia, 12-month prevalence estimates of partner abuse have varied from as low as 2.1% in a community crime victim survey[72] to as high as 28% in a general practice sample.[73] Such variations may reflect differences in the true prevalence of abuse from one sample to another. However, it is more likely that much of the discrepancy in prevalence rates is due to differences in definitions of partner abuse used by the researchers. The lower figures are obtained when IPV is classified as criminal assault by a partner in the home and the higher figures when a broader definition that includes infrequent minor physical abuse, sexual abuse, and emotional abuse is used.

In this detailed review, the methodologies of the prevalence studies of the most significant community samples, undertaken in English-speaking countries during the 1990s, will be reviewed. The aim is to highlight some methodological issues in the field of partner abuse research and in particular to explore the impact of different definitions of abuse on the findings of each study. Sample sizes, response rates, sample types, definitions of domestic violence used, questionnaire used, lifetime prevalence, and/or 12-month prevalence are compared. Data on male victims are included from studies in which it has been collected.

Community surveys

The majority of these studies were carried out in the mid-1980s to mid-1990s and generally have utilized the CTS or an adapted form of the CTS. Table 2.2 outlines some of these community studies, undertaken in English-speaking countries, with the main criteria for inclusion being the size of the sample. The most recent survey shown utilized an adapted form of the CTS to interview 6,300 women randomly drawn from the Australian electoral roll.[74] The definition of violence used in this study was based on actions, which could be considered as offences under State criminal law. The study found that 2.6% of women who were currently married or in a de facto relationship had experienced an incident of violence by their partner in the previous 12-month period and 8.0% at some stage in their relationship. The majority of this violence occurred only once (49.8%) or occurred rarely (26.2%) with the remainder occurring often (7.4%) or sometimes (16.5%). However, 42.4% of women who had had a previous relationship reported violence by a previous partner. Overall, 22.5% of women who currently or had ever had a partner had experienced physical violence. This last figure is similar to all other figures that use single physical acts (e.g. CTS violence items) as their measure of partner abuse. The use of the CTS has been widespread and community surveys utilizing this measure to date have uniformly resulted in figures of one in five to one in four lifetime prevalence of partner abuse.[52–55,72,74,75,77]

Table 2.2   Prevalence of IPA in selected community studies using national random samples

Year, country, first author	Sample size (response rate)	Definition used[a]	12–month prevalence (%)	Lifetime prevalence (%)
1986 USA Straus[53]	3,520 couples (84%)	Physical abuse Severe (kicked, bitten, or hit with a fist, hit or tried to hit with something, beat up, threatened with, or use of, knife or gun)	11.6 3.4	28.0 of couples
1987 Canada Smith[54]	604 women (56.4%)	Physical abuse Severe (as above)	14.4 5.1	25.0 7.1
1988 New Zealand Mullen[77]	1,516 women (73.9%)	Physical abuse 'hit and physically abused' 'hit and physically abused >3 times'	NA[b]	16.2 9.6
1992 Australia Ferrante[72]	1,511 men 1,550 women (52.7%)	'attacked, hit, pulled, pushed or punched in an aggressive or threatening manner' and stealing by threat or force, personal attack, threat with force, and sexual assault	2.1 women 0.2 men	NA
1994 Canada Rodgers[55]	12,300 women (67.0%)	Physical abuse (CTS)[c] Sexual assault	3.0	29.0 8.0
1996 Australia McLennan[74]	6,300 women (78%)	Physical violence (adapted CTS) Sexual violence (sexual assault/threat) Emotional abuse (insulted with intention to humiliate, damaged property, prevented access to money, car, telephone, family, friends, threatened children or pets)	NA 0.3[d] NA	22.5 1.0[d] 8.8[d]

[a] Unless otherwise stated, frequency of abuse is at east once.
[b] Not available.
[c] Conflict Tactics Scale.
[d] Of women in current relationships.

Crime victimization surveys

Some crime victimization studies have examined the frequency of assault in intimate relationships. An example of a comprehensive review using multiple sources of information to estimate the incidence and prevalence of domestic violence highlights the definitional issues. This study was conducted in Western Australia in 1995. It revealed incidence figures (estimated annual rates per 100,000 adult females) of domestic violence injury varying from as low as 1.6 (police-recorded homicides) to 129.2 (hospital admissions data), to 183.5 (recorded crime), to 248.1 (restraining order data), to 3,700 or 3.7% (survey data).[72] The corresponding 12-month prevalence figure for the crime victim survey of 1550 women was 2.1% (Table 2.2). If only acts involving injury were included in the definition then the prevalence dropped to 1%. All definitions in the context of crime victim surveys have resulted in much lower rates than community surveys utilizing the CTS physical items. Ferrante[72] has suggested that lower prevalence rates are obtained if one is researching physical violence as a crime, rather than in research where physical violence is seen as part of the spectrum of partner abuse.

Clinical studies

Many clinical studies have suffered from problems with definitional clarity and have tried to broaden the definitions used in the crime victimization surveys to include emotional abuse. To achieve this, most of the studies have used an adapted form of the CTS as their instrument. The researchers have included a combination of physical items from the CTS, and sexual and emotional abuse questions, constructed by the individual researcher and not validated. In practice, patients were defined as victims in these studies if they said 'yes' to one of the physical abuse items from the CTS or to the question 'Have you experienced emotional abuse?', and no estimation of the frequency of the acts was made in the majority of the studies (see Table 2.3). There is once again a striking similarity in the prevalence of physical abuse found across most of the studies of around one in four women.

Utilizing general questions, rather than specific questions about acts of abuse, may result in higher rates of abuse being reported. An emergency department survey utilized a general definition of abuse and obtained a very high lifetime prevalence rate of 54.2%.[78] Included in their definition of abuse were any patients who answered 'yes or unsure' to being 'threatened or physically injured at some time in their lives'.

General practice studies

General practice (GP) studies display a variation in prevalence depending on the definition and methodology used by each researcher. One Australian GP study obtained a very high 12-month prevalence rate of physical or emotional abuse of 28% of women who are in current relationships.[73] This rate is similar to the lifetime prevalence rates of other clinical studies using similar methodologies (Table 2.4). The figure is similar to two non-random, smaller GP studies.[32,81] A larger USA study ($n = 1,952$) obtained a much lower 12-month prevalence partner abuse rate of 5.5% of all women attending at four family practice clinics.[82] More recent larger GP studies in Australia, the USA, the UK, and Ireland have found high lifetime physical abuse rates ranging from 23.3 to 41.0% of women[60,83–85] and 12-month rates similar to the USA study.[82]

Methodological issues in IPA prevalence research

The above sections have described the problems with the existing measures of partner abuse and the partly related difficulties with definitional issues. In addition, there are other methodological challenges in any research on

Table 2.3   Prevalence of partner abuse in selected clinical studies

Year, country, first author	Sample size (response rate)	Sample type	Definition used[a]	12-month prevalence (%)	Lifetime prevalence (%)
1994 Australia Webster[79]	1,127 women (90%)	Consecutive patients at antenatal clinic	Physical abuse Sexual abuse Emotional abuse	NA[b]	23.0 5.3 21.2
1994 Australia Roberts[34]	1,326 men 1,110 women (67.7%)	Consecutive patients at emergency department	Physical abuse 'persistent abuse, with one partner being afraid of and/or being hurt by the other' Sexual abuse (not defined) Emotional abuse (verbal abuse, not allowed money, kept from family/friends)	2.7 men 7.4 women	8.8 men 23.6 women 6.9 19.2
1995 USA Abbott[78]	648 women (78%)	Consecutive patients at emergency department	'threatened or physically injured at some time in their lives' (patients who answered unsure were included as abused)	NA	54.2
1996 Australia de Vries Robbe[80]	475 men 522 women (97%)	Consecutive patients at emergency department	'persistent abuse, with one partner being afraid of and/or being hurt by the other'	2.9 men 7.1 women	8.5 men 19.3 women

[a]Unless otherwise stated, frequency of abuse is at least once.
[b]Not available.

Table 2.4 Prevalence of partner abuse in selected GP clinical studies

Year, country, first author	Sample size (response rate)	Sample type	Definition used[a]	12-month prevalence (%)	Lifetime prevalence (%)
1989 USA Rath[81]	218 women (not stated)	Non-random patients at 2 family practices	Verbal abuse		48.0
			Physical abuse minor (pushed or shoved)		44.0
			Physical abuse severe (hitting with fist, kicking)		28.0
1992 USA Hamberger[332]	476 women (not stated)	Consecutive patients at 1 family practice	Physical abuse (at least pushed or shoved)	23.0	38.0
1996 Australia Mazza[73]	2,181 women (72%)	Consecutive patients at 15 general practices	Physical abuse minor	22.0	NA
			Physical abuse severe	10.0	
			Emotional abuse (withheld money, prevented leaving home/seeing family, humiliated, threatened to kill)	20.0	
			Physical or emotional abuse	28.0[b]	
			Sexual abuse (rape, attempted rape) adapted CTS	13.0	
1996 USA McCauley[82]	1,952 women (66.9%)	Consecutive 4 patients at family practices	Physical abuse or sexual abuse (forced to have sexual activities) (adapted CTS)	5.5	21.4
2000 USA Coker[83]	1,401 women	Consecutive patients at 2 family practices	Total abuse		55.1
			Physical abuse		37.6
			Sexual abuse		19.5
			Index of spouse abuse		
2001 Ireland Bradley[85]	1,871 (72%)	Consecutive patients at 22 general practices	Physical abuse		39.0
			Emotional abuse (controlling behaviour)		69.0
			Afraid of partner		28.0
2001 UK Richardson[884]	1,207 (55%)	Consecutive patients at 13 general practices	Physical abuse	17.0	41.0
			Emotional abuse (controlling behaviour)		74.0
			Afraid of partner		35.0
2002 Australia Hegarty[60]	1,896 (78.5%)	Consecutive patients at 20 general practices	Total abuse	8.0	37.0
			Physical abuse	5.0	23.3
			Sexual abuse	1.9	10.6
			Emotional abuse	7.6	33.9
			Afraid of partner		28.0

[a]Unless otherwise stated frequency of abuse is at least once.
[b]CR is current relationships.

the prevalence of domestic violence. All survey-based abuse rates are likely to be underestimates of actual rates because of the likelihood of victims not to report abuse.[86] This may have several causes, which include social desirability, discrepant perception, and the potential impact of trauma if the abuse is recalled.[58,87]

A second issue is that of faulty recall, where victims may remember incidents as occurring more recently than they actually did. This 'forward telescoping' would inflate 12-month prevalence rates.[54] Alternatively, victims may 'backward telescope' events to reduce the prevalence rates. There also appears to be an effect on disclosure of abuse depending on the timing and format of the questions. In one study, an additional 10% of abused women were detected by an open supplementary question to the CTS, which asked about general abuse.[54] McFarlane[88] compared self-report questionnaires with nurse interview and found that self-report abuse by women on a standard medical history intake form revealed a lower prevalence (8%) than when they were asked the same abuse assessment questions by a health care provider (29%). In contrast, another study[89] found that subjects reported lower levels of violence during an in-depth interview than on a self-report questionnaire. Despite the problems with self-report, the survey remains the most pragmatic method of assessment of the prevalence of partner abuse.

CONCLUSION

This chapter has employed existing sources of data to review the nature of IPA and the methods used to estimate prevalence. There is strong evidence that IPA is a major public health problem with significant morbidity and mortality (see Chapter 3). The variations in prevalence found across studies might be due to a range of methodological problems, as well as genuine geographical and cultural variation. These problems include the source of the sample (clinical or community); the method of survey (self-report, telephone, or interview); the effect of faulty recall; and the potential impact of trauma if the abuse is recalled. However, the studies reviewed in this chapter have highlighted that, in spite of the lack of clarity about definitions, IPA is a very common, hidden problem for women attending clinical practice. Conservative estimates are that up to 1 in 10 women attending clinical practice are currently suffering persistent emotional, physical, and sexual abuse in an adult intimate relationship and one in five women suffer occasional physical abuse at the hands of their partners. A full-time primary care clinician is probably seeing at least one currently abused woman each week, although she may not be presenting with obvious signs or symptoms.[90] On average, 1 in 50 women are presenting to the emergency department because of IPA.[34]

For future research, we need to improve the operationalized definition that is used in the measurement of partner abuse; a definition where IPA is seen as a complex behavioural phenomenon that incorporates severity, frequency, meaning, and intention of any physical, emotional, and sexual act against a partner. Which relationships are included in estimates of prevalence should be clearly outlined; that is, women in current relationships only; women who have ever been in an intimate relationship; all women, heterosexual and homosexual; cohabiters and boyfriends/girlfriends. Finally, partner abuse against women is not just criminal assault in the home nor is it one isolated push or shove in a lifetime of a relationship, nor is it one episode of not being able to contact friends or family. Partner abuse is best understood as a chronic syndrome that is characterized not by episodes of violence but by the emotional and psychological abuse that is used by men to control their female partner.[10]

REFERENCES

1. Hegarty K, Roberts G. How common is domestic violence against women? The definition of partner abuse in prevalence studies. Aust N Z J Public Health 1998; 22:55–60.
2. Saltzman LE, et al. Intimate partner violence surveillance: uniform definitions and recommended data elements, Version 1.0. Atlanta: Centers for Disease Control and Prevention; 2002.
3. Krug EG, et al. World report on violence and health. Geneva: World Health Organization; 2002.
4. Candib LM. Violence against women: no more excuses. Fam Med 1989; 21(5):339–341.
5. Warshaw C. Limitations of the medical model in the care of battered women. Gend Soc 1989; 3(4):506–517.
6. Taft A. To screen or not to screen – is this the right question? Quality care, intervention and women's agency in health care responses to partner violence and abuse. Wom against Viol 2001; 10:41–46.
7. Yllo K. Through a feminist lens: gender, power and violence. In: Gelles RJ, Loseke DR, eds. Current controversies on family violence. Newbury Park, CA: Sage; 1993:47–63.
8. Watts C, Watts ZC. Violence against women: global scope and magnitude. Lancet 2002; 359:1232–1237.
9. Straus MA, Gelles RJ, Steinmetz SK. Behind closed doors: violence in the American family. New York: Doubleday/Anchor; 1980.
10. Sassetti MR. Domestic violence. Primary Care 1993; 20(2):289–304.
11. Follingstad DR, Rutledge LL, Berg BJ, et al. The role of emotional abuse in physically abusive relationships. J Fam Violence 1990; 5(2):107–120.
12. Marshall L. Effects of men's subtle and overt psychological abuse on low-income women. Violence Vict 1999; 14(1):69–88.
13. Okun L. Woman abuse: facts replacing myths. Albany, NY: SUNY Press; 1986.
14. DeKeseredy W, Hinch R. Woman abuse: sociological perspectives. Toronto: Thompson Educational; 1991.
15. Alexander R. Wife-battering: an Australian perspective. J Fam Violence 1993; 8(3):229–251.
16. Domestic violence. Australian Public Health Association; 1990.
17. Dobash RP, Dobash RE. Violence against wives: a case against the patriarchy. New York: Free Press; 1979.
18. Johnson MP. Patriarchal terrorism and common couple violence: two forms of violence against women. J Marriage Fam 1995; 57:283–294.
19. Neidig PH, Freidman DH. Spouse abuse: a treatment program for couples. Introduction to the program. Illinois: Research Press; 1984:1–25.
20. Johnson PJ, Hellerstedt WL, Pirie PL. Abuse history and nonoptimal prenatal weight gain. Public Health Reports 2002; 117(2):148–156.
21. Community attitudes of violence against women. Canberra: ANOP Research Services; 1995.
22. Domestic violence in Australia. Office of the Status of Women. Canberra: Elliot and Shanahan Research; 1988.
23. Mugford J. Violence today, No.2: Domestic violence. Canberra: National Committee on Violence; 1989.
24. Goodman L, Koss M, Fitzgerald L, et al. Male violence against women: current research and future directions. American Psychologist 1993; 48(10):1054–1058.

25. Dobash R, Dobash RP. Women, violence and social change. London: Routledge; 1992:251–283.
26. Gelles R, Straus M. Intimate violence: the causes and consequences of abuse in the American family. New York: Rockefeller; 1988.
27. Head C, Taft A. Improving general practitioner management of women experiencing domestic violence: a study of the beliefs and experiences of women victim/survivors and of GPs. Canberra: Department of Health, Housing and Community Service; 1995.
28. Hotaling GT, Sugarman DB. An analysis of risk markers in husband to wife violence: the current state of knowledge. Violence Vict 1986; 1(2):101–124.
29. Doumas D, Margolin G, John R. The intergenerational transmission of aggression across three generations. J Fam Violence 1994; 10:157–175.
30. Gelles RJ. Physical violence, child abuse, and child homicide: a continuum of violence or distinct behaviors. Hum Nat 1991; 2(1):59–72.
31. Bergman BK, Brismar BG. Can family violence be prevented? A psychosocial study of male batterers and battered wives. Public Health 1992; 106:45–52.
32. Hamberger LK, Saunders DG, Hovey M. Prevalence of domestic violence in community practice and rate of physician inquiry. Fam Med 1992; 24:283–287.
33. American Public Health Association. Domestic violence. Am J Public Health 1993; 83(3):458–463.
34. Roberts G, O'Toole B, Lawrence J, et al. Domestic violence victims in a hospital emergency department. Med J Aust 1994; 159:307–310.
35. Smith J, Williams J. From abusive household to dating violence. J Fam Violence 1992; 11:153–165.
36. Straus MA. Measuring intrafamily conflict and violence: the Conflict Tactics (CT) Scale. J Marriage Fam 1979; February:75–79.
37. Gelles RJ. Through a sociological lens. In: Gelles RJ, Loseke DR, eds. Current controversies in family violence. Newbury Park, CA: Sage; 1993:31–47.
38. Finkelhor D. Common features of family abuse. In: Finkelhor D, Gelles R, Hotaling G, et al., eds. The dark side of families: current family violence research. Newbury Park, CA; Sage: 1983.
39. Anderson ML. Thinking about women: sociological perspectives on sex and gender, 3rd edn. New York: Macmillan; 1993.
40. Dobash RE, Dobash RP. Research as social action: the struggle for battered women. In: Yllo K, Bograd M, eds. Feminist perspectives on wife abuse. Newbury Park, CA: Sage; 1988:51–74.
41. Stark E, Flitcraft A. Violence among intimates: an epidemiological review. In: Van Hasselt VB, Morrison RL, Bellack AS, et al., eds. Handbook of family violence. New York: Plenum Press; 1988:293–316.
42. Koss MP. Deleterious effects of criminal victimisation on women's health and medical utilisation. Arch Intern Med 1991; 151:342–347.
43. Bograd M. Feminist perspectives on wife abuse: an introduction. In: Yllo K, Bograd M, eds. Feminist perspectives on wife abuse. Newbury Park, CA: Sage; 1988: 11–25.
44. Coleman KH, Weinman ML, His BP. Factors affecting conjugal violence. J Psychol 1980; 105:97–102.
45. Hoff LA. Collaborative feminist research and the myth of objectivity. In: Yllo K, Bograd M, eds. Feminist perspectives on wife abuse. Newbury Park, CA: Sage; 1988:269–281.
46. Sugarman DB, Frankel SL. Patriarchal ideology and wife-assault: a meta-analytic review. J Fam Violence 1996; 11(1):13–40.
47. Straus MA. The Conflict Tactics Scale and its critics: an evaluation and new data on validity and reliability, in physical violence. In: Straus MA, Gelles RJ, eds. American families: risk factors and adaptions to violence in 8,145 families. New Brunswick: Transaction Publishers; 1990:49–75.
48. Candib LM. Naming the contradiction: family medicine's failure to face violence against women. Fam Community Health 1990; 13(3):47–57.
49. Rose K, Saunders DG. Nurses and physicians attitudes about women abuse: the effects of gender and professional role. Health Care Women Int 1986; 7:427–438.

50. Tolman R. The development of a measure of psychological maltreatment of women by their male partners. Violence Vict 1989; 4(3):159–177.

51. Walker LE. The battered woman. New York: Harper and Row; 1979.

52. O'Leary KD. Through a psychological lens: personality traits, personality disorders, and levels of violence. In: Gelles RJ, Loseke DR, eds. Current controversies in family violence. Newbury Park, CA: Sage; 1993:7–31.

53. Straus MA, Gelles RJ. Societal change and change in family violence from 1975 to 1985 as revealed by two national surveys. J Marriage Fam 1986; 48(August):465–479.

54. Smith M. The incidence and prevalence of woman abuse in Toronto. Violence Vict 1987; 2:173–187.

55. Rodgers K. Wife assault: the findings of a national survey. Statistics Canada Catalogue 1994; 14(9):1–21.

56. Koss M. The women's mental health research agenda. Am Psychol 1990; 45(3):374–380.

57. Saunders DG. Wife abuse, husband abuse or mutual combat: a feminist perspective on the empirical findings. In: Yllo K, Bograd M, eds. Feminist perspectives on wife abuse. Newbury Park, CA: Sage; 1988:91–113.

58. DeKeseredy WS. Enhancing the quality of survey data on woman abuse: examples from a national Canadian study. Violence Against Women 1995; 1(2):158–173.

59. Hegarty KL, Sheehan M, Schonfeld C. A multidimensional definition of partner abuse: development and preliminary validation of the Composite Abuse Scale. J Fam Violence 1999; 14(4):399–414.

60. Hegarty K, Bush R. Prevalence of partner abuse in women attending Australian General Practice: a cross-sectional survey. Aust N Z J Public Health 2002; 26(5):437–442.

61. Loring MT. Emotional abuse. New York: Lexington; 1994.

62. Straus MA, Hamby SL, Boney-McCoy S, et al. The Revised Conflicts Tactics Scale (CTS2) development and preliminary psychometric data. J Fam Issues 1996; 17(3):283–316.

63. Statulevicius E. Measuring incidence of domestic violence: an investigation of gender differences and methodologically flawed research. Queensland: University of Queensland; 1991.

64. Rodenberg F, Fantuzzo J. The measure of wife abuse: steps toward the development of a comprehensive assessment technique. J Fam Violence 1993; 8(3):203–217.

65. Margolin G, Sibner L, Glegerman L. Wife battering. In: Van Hasselt VB, Morrison RL, Bellack AS, et al., eds. Handbook of family violence. New York: Plenum Press; 1988:89–117.

66. Hudson W, McIntosh S. The assessment of spouse abuse: two quantifiable dimensions. J Marriage Fam 1981; 43:873–888.

67. Shepard MF, Campbell JA. The abusive behavior inventory: a measure of psychological and physical abuse. J Interpers Violence 1992; 7(3):291–305.

68. Hegarty K, Bush R, Sheahan M. The Composite Abuse Scale: further development and assessment of reliability in two clinical settings. Violence Vict 2004. In press.

69. Marshall L. Development of the Severity of Violence Against Women Scales. J Fam Violence 1992; 7(2):103–121.

70. Geffner R, Rosenbaum A, Hughes H. Research issues concerning family violence. In: Van Hasselt VB, Morrison RL, Bellack AS, et al., eds. Handbook of family violence. New York: Plenum Press; 1988:457–481.

71. Heise L. Violence against women: the hidden health burden. WHO Health Statistics Quarterly, 1993; 46:78–85.

72. Ferrante A, Indermaur D, Morgan F, et al. Measuring the extent of domestic violence. Sydney: Hawkins Press; 1996.

73. Mazza D, Dennerstein L, Ryan V. Physical, sexual and emotional violence against women: a general practice-based prevalence study. Med J Aust 1996; 164:14–17.

74. McLennan W. Women's Safety Survey. Canberra: Australian Bureau of Statistics; 1996.

75. Ratner P. The incidence of wife abuse and mental health status in abused wives in Edmonton, Alberta. Can J Public Health 1993; 84(4):246–249.

76. DeKeseredy W, Kelly K. The incidence and prevalence of woman abuse in Canadian university and college dating relationships. Can J Sociol 1993; 18(2):137–156.

77. Mullen P, Walton V, Romans-Clarkson S, et al. Impact of sexual and physical abuse on women's mental health. Lancet 1988; (April 16):841–845.
78. Abbott J, Johnson R, Koziol-McLain J, et al. Domestic violence against women: incidence and prevalence in an emergency department population. JAMA 1995; 273(22):1763–1767.
79. Webster J, Sweett S, Stolz TA. Domestic violence in pregnancy: a prevalence study. Med J Aust 1994; 161(8):466–470.
80. de Vries Robbe M, March L, Vinen J, et al. Prevalence of domestic violence among patients attending a hospital emergency department. Aust N Z J Public Health 1996; 20(4):364–368.
81. Rath GD, Jaratt LG, Leonardson G. Rates of domestic violence against adult women by men partners. J Am Board Fam Prac 1989; 2:227–233.
82. McCauley J, Kern DE, Kolodner K, et al. The 'battering syndrome': prevalence and clinical characteristics of domestic violence in primary care internal medicine practices. Ann Intern Med 1995; 123:737–746.
83. Coker AL. Frequency and correlates of intimate partner violence by type: physical, sexual and psychological battering. Am J Public Health 2000; 90(4):553–559.
84. Richardson J, Coid J, Petruckevitch A, et al. Identifying domestic violence: cross sectional study in primary care. Brit Med J 2002; 324:1–6.
85. Bradley F, et al. Reported frequency of domestic violence: cross sectional survey of women attending general practice. Brit Med J 2002; 324:1–6.
86. Arias I, Beach SR. Validity of self reports of marital violence. J Fam Violence 1987; 2(2):139–149.
87. Smith MD. Enhancing the quality of survey data on violence against women: a feminist approach. Gend Soc 1994; 18:19–127.
88. McFarlane J, Christoffel K, Bateman L, et al. Assessing for abuse: self-report versus nurse interview. Public Health Nurs 1991; 8(4):245–250.
89. Rhodes N. The assessment of spousal abuse: an alternative to the Conflict Tactics Scale. In: Viano EC, ed. Intimate violence: interdisciplinary perspectives. San Francisco: Hemisphere Publishing; 1992.
90. Hegarty KL. Measuring a multidimensional definition of domestic violence: prevalence of partner abuse in women attending general practice. Unpublished doctoral thesis. Brisbane: University of Queensland; 1999.

SECTION 2

Impact, education, identification, and intervention

Chapter **3**

Impact of intimate partner abuse on physical and mental health: how does it present in clinical practice?

Jacquelyn C Campbell, Kathryn Laughon, and Anne Woods

I mean words hurt me [and] the physical part, hurt too. This [injury] hurt, yes, but the words, calling me . . . no good, and just different stuff, that hurt me, too. It makes your self-esteem not really good. I didn't feel good about myself.
42-year-old survivor of intimate partner abuse

INTRODUCTION

Women who experience Intimate Partner Abuse (IPA) are significantly more likely to experience physical and psychological symptoms and to seek health care for stress-related and chronic ailments than non-abused women.[1,2] Recent research demonstrates that intimate partner violence (IPV) and abuse are very common in women presenting to emergency departments (past-year prevalence: 15–18%; lifetime prevalence: 37–50%),[3,4,5] primary care clinics (past-year prevalence: 8–29%; lifetime prevalence: 20–51%),[6,7,8,14] and obstetric/gynaecologic services (6–21% during pregnancy; 13–21% postpartum).[9,10,11,12] In addition, 41% of women who were killed by an intimate partner in the United States utilized health care agencies for injury or physical or mental health problems in the year prior to femicide.[13] Identifying women who are experiencing, or have a history of, IPA and IPV in the clinical setting presents the opportunity for intervention, but recognition of these conditions is challenging and complex. This chapter will address how IPA and IPV present in various health care settings based on evidence from recent research. Clinical indicators of IPA and suggestions of mechanisms that may explain its presentation will also be discussed. We will use a definition of IPV condensed from that developed by a consensus panel for the US Centers for Disease Control and Prevention (CDC) as follows: physical and/or sexual assault or threats of assault against a married, cohabitating, or dating current or estranged intimate partner by the other partner, also including emotional abuse and controlling behaviours in a relationship where there has been physical and/or sexual assault.[14] (See Chapter 2.) The term IPA will be used when the abuse being measured included emotional abuse and controlling behaviours.

Women seldom present with a chief complaint of partner abuse, and rates of inquiry by health care professionals about abuse vary depending on the site of care, the health care provider, and the type of visit (see Chapter 5). Among women seen in general practice settings, 8% self-reported IPV and only 12–20% of those victimized reported that their physician asked about partner abuse.[7,15] Within emergency room settings across 11 mid-sized community-level hospitals in Pennsylvania and California, fewer than 25% of women stated that they were asked about IPA by the clinical staff. This inquiry rate was higher for women with acute trauma (39%) than for women who had been abused in the last year (13%). However, 76% of women experiencing IPA within the past year and more than one-third of those who recently experienced IPA did not present to the emergency department for treatment of an injury but for other reasons such as an acute illness.[16] Complicating the picture is the lack of a convenient way to assess who is at increased risk for IPA. Although women are more at risk if they are of a younger age, divorced or separated, poorer, or have been previously traumatized, there is no risk factor that is particularly strong or any combination that is consistent.[17,18,19,20,21] All women are at some risk for abuse by an intimate partner and battered women may present in any health care setting. Therefore, it is particularly important to understand the clinical presentations for which or with which they may seek health care.

PHYSICAL HEALTH CONSEQUENCES OF IPV

IPV has significant negative physical health consequences. Perhaps the most obvious is physical injury, with fractures, lacerations, contusions, and tendon or ligament damage to the face, neck, upper torso, breast, or abdomen being most common.[22,23,24,25,26] At least half of women who experience IPV are injured by the abuse,[11,18] and intimate partners are responsible for 30% of female homicides in the United States.[27] Short-term sequelae consist of pain and decreased function related to the traumatic injury.

The effects of IPV may also result in less obvious, long-term physical health sequelae. Coker and colleagues' population-based study utilizing the National Violence Against Women Survey in the United States found that physical IPV was significantly associated with developing a chronic physical health condition (adjusted relative risk = 1.6, 95% confidence interval (CI) = 1.3–2.0) and women reported that this interfered with normal activities in the past week.[2] A recent large case-control study of enrollees in a multisite metropolitan health maintenance organization found that abused women had approximately a 60% higher rate of all physical health problems in the past year compared to never abused women (incidence rate ratio = 1.58, 95% CI = 1.34–1.86; $p < 0.001$), even though the abuse could have occurred as long as eight years prior to the study.[1] These long-term sequelae can present as central nervous system problems such as seizures related to head injury; musculoskeletal problems such as arthritis or chronic back pain; gynaecological symptoms such as sexually transmitted infections (STIs), vaginal bleeding, vaginal infection, chronic pelvic pain, dyspareunia, and urinary tract infections; conditions associated with chronic stress, such as headaches, hypertension, cardiac problems, loss of appetite, abdominal pain, or digestive problems; and immune system alterations, such as asthma, allergies, rash, diabetes, upper respiratory infections, and cancer.[1,2] These studies support a substantial body of research documenting significantly impaired physical health in women who survive IPV compared to non-abused women.[28,29,30,31,32,33,34,35,36] What is not known for sure is what percentage of these symptoms and conditions are related to old injuries, perhaps inadequately diagnosed and/or treated, and what proportion are related to other mechanisms, such as the type of abuse or stress and its effects on various physiological mechanisms.

Sexually transmitted infections

STIs represent an important source of morbidity among the women at highest risk for IPV (poor, minority women of childbearing age) and they merit particular discussion. In the United States, the Centers for Disease Control and Prevention found that in 2001, the rates of chlamydia and gonorrhoea were, respectively, 435 and 125 per 100,000 among adult women. The risk of STIs among abused women is 2–4 times that of non-abused women. A population-based study found that 41.1% of abused women vs. 9.0% of non-abused women had an STI in the past five years.[37] A two-year longitudinal study found that the risk of STIs among abused women was just over four times higher than for non-abused women when they first joined the study and just under at two years (4.3 vs. 3.8).[38] Coker et al. found that invasive cervical neoplasia (most often caused by the sexually transmitted human papillomavirus) was four times more common among sexually abused women.[39] (Human papillomavirus, an STI, is the primary cause of cervical neoplasia.[40]) The research in this area provides moderate evidence of a relationship between abuse and increased risk of a variety of STIs in the mostly poor, mostly minority populations studied in the United States. The generalizability of these findings is hindered by use of convenience samples (mostly in clinic populations) and their use of poor, mostly ethnic minority women in the United States. The cross-sectional design of most of the studies precludes drawing conclusions about the causal relationships between violence and disease.

It is important to note, however, that these findings most likely underestimated STI prevalence since most relied on self-report. Women may have been reluctant to disclose STIs to researchers. Additionally, many STIs can be asymptomatic and the infections therefore undiagnosed. (The Institute of Medicine in the US estimates that diagnosed cases of chlamydia and gonorrhoea represent only 50% of actual cases, a finding supported by recent research.[41,42]) It is therefore reasonable to imagine that the incidence of both IPV and STIs in these studies are even higher than reported. Abuse was probably also underestimated in these studies. Many of the studies used non-specific questions such as 'Have you been abused?', which result in lower rates of detection than more specific questions. (See Chapter 2.)

The causes of increased incidence of STIs among women experiencing IPV are not known, although a number of plausible mechanisms have been proposed. Forced sex occurs in approximately 40–45% of physically violent intimate relationships[43] and is associated with a 2–10 times higher risk of STIs than physical abuse alone.[39,44,45,46] Forced sex may cause genital injuries that facilitate disease transmission.[38]

Findings from both qualitative and quantitative studies indicate that condom use is more difficult to negotiate in violent relationships.[45,47,48,49,50,51,52,53] Although several small studies have found that abused women use condoms at the same rate as non-abused women,[54,55] the preponderance of the research findings indicate less condom use among abused women.

A number of researchers have examined the relationship between high-risk sexual behaviour (other than intercourse without condoms) and current or past IPA. Behaviours examined varied from study to study and included: multiple sexual partners, sex in exchange for money or drugs, and having sex with high-risk partners.[47,49,53,55,56,57,58,59] Findings from all of these studies, albeit all using small convenience samples from US populations and cross-sectional designs, indicated a relationship between a variety of high-risk sexual behaviours and IPA. Interestingly, one study also found more high-risk behaviours among men who had abused a female partner in the past year compared to men without such a history.[60] A dose–response relationship between severity of IPV and degree of physical health problems has also been demonstrated, but even women experiencing low-severity violence report significantly increased symptoms.[61]

The childbearing year

During the childbearing period, women are at special risk for IPV with serious sequelae for mother and child (see Chapter 7). Janssen and colleagues found a significantly increased risk for antepartum haemorrhage (adjusted odds ratio = 3.79, 95% CI = 1.38–10.4), intrauterine growth restriction (odds ratio = 3.06, 95% CI = 1.02–9.14), and perinatal death (odds ratio = 8.06, 95% CI = 1.42–45.63).[62] Several studies also document an association of IPV with abortion, miscarriage, abruptio placenta, low birthweight (LBW), preterm labour, and caesarean section.[63,64,65,66,67] A recent meta-analysis of abuse during pregnancy and birthweight found a significant association across studies in the US and Canada.[68]

Women are also at increased risk for IPV-related femicide during the childbearing year. In a groundbreaking case control study across 10 cities in the United States, McFarlane and her colleagues found femicide to be a significant cause of maternal mortality. Among 437 cases of attempted/completed femicide, 5% of victims were murdered while pregnant. The risk of attempted or completed femicide was three times higher for women abused during pregnancy (adjusted odds ratio = 3.08, 95% CI = 2.4–5.5) than for women who were abused but not during pregnancy. Black women were at even greater risk than white women.[69]

The infant remains at risk even after delivery. McFarlane and Soeken found that among an ethnically stratified cohort of 121 women who experienced IPV during pregnancy, weight gain from 6 to 12 months was less in infants where abuse continued after 6 months.[70] Additionally, the risk of child abuse may be particularly severe when abuse occurred during pregnancy, with a significant association of child abuse and IPA shown in several studies.[71] This indicates a need for multidisciplinary attention to risk factors for IPA within paediatric settings.

Overall health

Living with IPV has immediate as well as long-lasting effects on women's physical health that results in abused women having a significantly poorer perception of their overall health, a greater number of physical health problems, and an increased use of emergency room services, general clinic visits, and hospitalizations compared to non-abused women.[1,2,72,73]

MENTAL HEALTH CONSEQUENCES OF IPA

Living in an abusive relationship also has significant effects on a woman's mental health status. For many women, abuse by an intimate partner is not comprised of a single episode, and 25–30% of abused women are cyclically beaten, many as often as once a week.[73] Emotional and sexual abuse frequently coexist with physical violence in a scenario of coercive control. Between 40 and 45% of physically abused women are subjected to forced sex or sexually degrading acts in the relationship.[10] A battered woman lives in realistic fear of further beatings, rape, injury, and possible death.

Structural factors within an abusive relationship may serve to mediate the relationship between IPA and mental health sequelae. Social isolation, lack of social support systems, restricted educational opportunities, job instability, and financial insecurity are significantly associated with poorer mental health symptoms.[74,75,76] Multiple mental health sequelae have been documented in abused women, including depression, post-traumatic stress disorder (PTSD), phobias, anxiety, panic disorders, and substance abuse disorders.[2,77,78,79,80] A comprehensive meta-analysis by Golding showed that, compared to rates in general populations of women, abused women had significantly greater mean weighted prevalence rates of depression (47.6%; weighted mean odds ratio = 3.8; 95% CI = 3.16–4.57), suicidality (17.0%; weighted mean odds = 1.4–4.59, depending on population), PTSD (63.8%, weighted mean odds = 3.74; 95% CI = 1.02–6.83); alcohol abuse (18.5%, weighted mean odds = 5.56; 90% CI = 3.32–9.31); and drug abuse (8.9%; weighed mean odds = 5.62; 95% CI = 3.55–7.72).[81] The studies drawn for this review were in both community and clinical settings. Two recent primary care studies have supported the strong link between depression and partner abuse for women attending general practitioners.[82,83] Depression in abused women has been associated with daily stressors, childhood abuse, forced sex in the relationship, marital separations, change in residence, negative life events, increased number of children, and child behaviour problems.[84,85] Factors contributing to PTSD include partner dominance, isolation, the degree of severity of physical violence, forced sex in the relationship, a history of child sexual abuse, and a greater mean number of traumas.[85,86,87,88,89] Longitudinal evidence suggests that while depression lessens with decreasing IPV, PTSD appears to be more persistent.[43] Among a community sample of 160 abused, post-abused, and non-abused women, up to 66% continued to have PTSD symptoms in spite of the fact that they had been out of the abusive relationship an average of 9 years (range = 2–23 years).[90] This finding is consistent with population-based studies of PTSD persistence.[91,92]

Examining depression and PTSD in women who are abused is complicated by the fact that PTSD is a complex disorder that frequently coexists with other mental health disorders. A greater number of empirical studies addressing the mental health effects of abuse address these comorbidities but fail to measure PTSD. One reason for this may be that patients typically do not approach the health care system complaining of PTSD, and primary care providers may not be attuned to a PTSD assessment and diagnosis. A small study that specifically examined the comorbidity of major depressive disorder and PTSD in abused women found that current IPV-related PTSD and depressive symptoms were strongly correlated ($r = 0.84$, $p < 0.001$), and that in 75% of cases, major depression occurred in the context of PTSD.[93] This correlation was confirmed in a large case control study of racially balanced, highly educated, middle-class working women, drawn from female health maintenance organization enrollees in a metropolitan city in the United States. There was a far greater prevalence of comorbid depressive/PTSD symptoms among women with a history of IPA (13.1%) than for pure depressive (4.6%) or PTSD (7.1%) symptoms alone. This comorbidity pattern also held true for controls in the study.[94]

Substance abuse is also a frequent comorbidity factor among abused women, with studies reporting significantly increased risk for alcohol, tobacco, recreational drugs, and prescription drug abuse.[2,61,78,81,95] Comorbidity results in more severe sequelae related to health, social functioning, and quality of life.[96,97] Golding[81] calculated a mean prevalence of alcohol abuse or dependence of 18.5% (95% CI = 15.9–21.3) and a mean prevalence of drug abuse or dependence of 8.9% (95% CI = 6.1–12.1) among abused women. A review article also found support for a link between IPA and use of substances.[98] A nationally representative sample of women in the US found that a history of physical and/or sexual assault (stranger and IPV) predicted alcohol dependence.[99] A number of smaller clinical and community convenience samples have also demonstrated a correlation between IPA and alcohol use.[100,101,102] Conversely, studies of substance-using women have shown higher rates of IPA than rates among non-substance-using women.[103,104]

A few studies have failed to find an association between substance use and IPA. One such study relied on chart review, making it difficult to ascertain how substance use had been assessed[105] and another did not include a non-abused control group.[106] Despite some conflicting findings, however, research supports increased prevalence of substance use among women with IPA.

The causes for the increased use of substances in this population of women have not been definitively proven, but some indicators are emerging. Findings from both longitudinal and cross-sectional studies using causal modelling techniques are beginning to support the notion that trauma precedes substance use, rather than the converse.[107,108,109,110] It is likely that major depressive disorder and PTSD mediate the relationship between trauma and substance use. One study has directly validated the role of PTSD as a mediator between childhood abuse and adult alcohol use.[111] Other researchers have demonstrated that PTSD precedes substance use, that the severity of PTSD is correlated with the severity of addiction, and that the types of PTSD symptoms are correlated with the type of addiction.[112] Findings from a longitudinal study of PTSD and drug use show that, while PTSD increased the risk of drug disorders after exposure to a traumatic event, substance use did not increase the risk of PTSD after a similar event.[113] A similar study found that having a PTSD diagnosis tripled the odds of a subsequent alcohol-related disorder.[114] Kilpatrick and colleagues'[99] population-based longitudinal analysis of the relationship between PTSD and substance use found that while *existing* substance use can lead to increased risk of trauma, and thus increased rates of PTSD, trauma and PTSD preceded the *first* use of substances. At least one study found that depression mediated the relationship between victimization and substance use.[110]

More work in this area is needed, but there is strong evidence from large probability samples to support a causal pathway from trauma to PTSD and subsequent substance use in women. The evidence of a relationship between depression and substance abuse is weaker, and is possibly explained by the strong degree of comorbidity between PTSD and depression in traumatized women.[115] It is interesting to note that the relationships among trauma, mental health disorders, and substance use is significantly stronger among women than among men.[110,116,117,118]

BIO–PSYCHO–SOCIO–IMMUNOLOGICAL MECHANISMS IN IPA

Women who experience IPA live with a combination of ongoing chronic stress and exacerbations of acute stress related to episodes of physical, psychological and sexual violence. Although the interrelatedness of stress and health has been recognized since ancient times, research establishing causal pathways between IPA and the multitude of physical and mental health effects is sparse. The complex relationships between women's experiences of abuse and poor physical and mental health outcomes point toward multiple causes.

Some of the physical health effects of IPA may be directly related to physical trauma. Neurological sequelae consisting of greater prevalence of headaches and seizures may be a direct result of head trauma or choking/incomplete strangulation that result in loss of consciousness.[119] Gastrointestinal disorders, which are consistently reported with greater frequency in abused women, may likewise be related to functional damage to the gastrointestinal tract subsequent to direct trauma, such as blows to the abdomen, or may be related to the effects of chronic stress and PTSD. Several researchers have demonstrated an association of irritable bowel syndrome with partner abuse and PTSD.[120,121,122]

The effects of stress on physical health are mediated by over-responsiveness of the autonomic nervous system or impaired immune system function; and there is strong support for the role of cortisol and catecholamines in this process.[123,124] Excessive secretion of these stress hormones in response to a perceived threat stimulate target organs. Organ dysfunction results when this stress response is not effectively modulated.

In addition to irritable bowel syndrome, there are numerous other examples of stress-related illnesses that are more commonly reported in abused women. Increased sympathetic nervous system activity that increases muscle contraction may result in tension headaches and lower back pain. Migraine headaches may also be a result of increased sympathetic response, with increased norepinephrine and serotonin levels causing vasoconstriction, which is responsible for the prodrome of an impending migraine, followed by rapid vasodilation and subsequent pain.

Cardiovascular conditions such as hypertension, chest pain, and palpitations have been strongly linked to sympathetic nervous system reactivity. Stress hormones elevate blood pressure in order to transport blood to areas where it is needed to engage in the classic 'fight or flight' reaction. In the presence of chronic stress, the increased alpha-adrenergic tone results in increased peripheral vascular resistance and sustained hypertension.

The increased reported prevalence of allergies, upper respiratory infections, STIs, and urinary tract infections may also be mediated through the complex interactions between the brain and body via direct and/or indirect effects on the central nervous system, immune system, or neuroendocrine–immune pathways. The effects of IPA on immune function may be related to differences in cortisol and cytokine levels, and subsequently on Th cell balance, that occur in relation to the mental health effects of violence, specifically depression and PTSD. Constantino and her colleagues recently demonstrated a significant correlation of depression and total mitogen response (a biological measure of decreased T-cell function) in abused women compared to non-abused women.[125] Unfortunately, there was potential confounding in that investigation due to tobacco use in all the abused women. In another small study, women with PTSD who had a history of childhood sexual trauma demonstrated a significant increase in biological markers for increased immune activation (CD45RO/CD45RA lymphocyte ratio) compared to matched controls.[126] These results are strengthened by greater control of confounding variables in that none of the subjects smoked, abused drugs or alcohol, or were pregnant or medically ill. Further effects on impaired immune system function in abused women are also likely mediated through the greater prevalence of substance use/abuse, including tobacco, alcohol, and drugs.

The numerous gynaecological problems found in battered women may be related to the increased risk of exposure to STIs due to refusal to use condoms, as well as to the direct trauma to the mucous membranes of the vagina, anus, and urethra during forced sex, leading to increased transmission of bacteria.

The effects of IPA on pregnancy outcomes are likely mediated via multiple pathways. The occurrence of abruptio placenta during pregnancy may be related to punches or kicks to the abdomen, as well as to the presence of hypertension or cocaine use, which is more prevalent in abused women. Intrauterine growth restriction and LBW may be associated with the physical health effects of violence, such as increased prevalence of hypertension or infections, as well as with the social effects of IPA, such as increased use of tobacco, alcohol, and drugs, or low maternal weight gain during pregnancy.[127,128] Preterm birth may be a result of STIs or urinary tract infections, or as a direct result of trauma. It is not known how the acute and chronic stress of living with IPA during pregnancy may affect neonatal outcomes. Animal studies demonstrate structural alterations in the newborn brain as well as alterations of the hypothalamic pituitary adrenal axis offspring of rodent mothers repeatedly stressed during gestation.[123]

Much remains to be done in investigating the causal pathways by which IPA affects women's health.

ADDRESSING IPA IN HEALTH CARE SETTINGS

Due to the high prevalence of IPA, its association with poorer physical and mental health, and the increased use of health care resources, it is reasonable to anticipate that all health care providers will come into contact with survivors of abuse. Since there are no convenient demographic indicators for IPA, clinicians must be alert to the clinical signs of abuse in all women. (See Table 3.1.) While signs of physical trauma may be most obvious, the majority of women will present with a constellation of possible and often intertwined physical and mental health problems. The presence of depressive and/or PTSD symptoms, substance abuse disorders, chronic pain, frequent infections, and frequent gynaecological disorders may serve as indicators for heightened suspicion of IPA. Conversely, if a woman says she is abused, the clinician should be alerted to her increased risk for a number of physical and mental health disorders as well as for the safety issues

Table 3.1 Signs of possible IPA on physical examination

Area of assessment	Findings indicating increased index of suspicion for IPA
General appearance	Increased anxiety in presence of spouse Signs of fatigue Inappropriate or anxious non-verbal behaviour Non-verbal communication suggesting shame about body Flinches when touched Poor grooming, inappropriate attire
Skin	Bruises, welts, oedema, or scars, especially if in various stages of healing and/or on breasts, upper arms, abdomen, chest, face, and genitalia Burns
Head	Subdural haematoma Clumps of hair missing
Eyes	Swelling Subconjunctival haemorrhage
Genital/urinary	Oedema, bruises, tenderness, external bleeding
Rectal	Bruising, bleeding, oedema, irritation
Musculoskeletal	Fractures, especially of facial bones, spiral fractures of radius or ulna, ribs Shoulder dislocation Limited motion of an extremity Old fractures in various stages of healing
Abdomen	Abdominal injuries in pregnant women Intra-abdominal injury
Neurological	Hyperactive reflex responses Ear or eye problems secondary to injury Areas of numbness from old injuries Tremors
Mental status examination	Anxiety, fear Depression Suicidal ideation Low self-esteem Memory loss Difficulty concentrating

related to domestic violence. Ideally, clinicians would then assess for sexually transmitted disease and mental health and substance use disorders. The occurrence of intrauterine growth restriction during pregnancy and LBW at delivery may also serve as potential alerts for IPA. It is imperative to continue assessing for IPA even after delivery, since the threat of femicide as a cause of maternal mortality is increased for women who are abused. It may be abused women who are more likely to miss postpartum visits, and these women would also be considered at high risk and therefore ideally a priority for postpartum home visitation. However, since all women are at risk of IPA, it is important that research be conducted to determine the feasibility, costs, and benefits of screening at all or certain specified visits for health care for all females. The most appropriate means for screening in specific settings, as well as who should do the screening and the interventions indicated, are currently being developed and tested (see Chapter 5). More research can also help determine the functional and physiological mechanisms by which abused women's health is compromised. Once identified, abused women can be offered referrals to domestic violence advocacy and programmes. It is extremely important that the health deficits that so commonly accompany IPA be identified and addressed.

REFERENCES

1. Campbell J, Jones AL, Dienemann J, et al. Intimate partner violence and physical health consequences. Arch Intern Med 2002; 162:1157–1163.
2. Coker AL, Davis KE, Arias I, et al. Physical and mental health effects of intimate partner violence for men and women. Am J Prev Med 2002; 23(4):260–268.
3. Dearwater SR, Coben JH, Campbell JC, et al. Prevalence of intimate partner abuse in women treated at community hospital emergency departments. JAMA 1998; 280(5):433–438.
4. El-Bassel N, Gilbert L, Witte S, et al. Intimate partner violence and substance abuse among minority women receiving care from an inner-city emergency department. Women Health Iss 2003; 13(1):16–22.
5. Ernst AA, Weiss SJ. Intimate partner violence from the emergency medicine perspective. Women Health 2002; 35(2–3):71–81.
6. Bauer HM, Rodriguez MA, Perez-Stable EJ. Prevalence and determinants of intimate partner abuse among public hospital primary care patients. J Gen Intern Med 2000; 15(11):811–817.
7. Hegarty KL, Bush R. Prevalence and associations of partner abuse in women attending general practice: a cross-sectional survey. Aust N Z J Public Health 2002; 26(5):437–442.
8. Naumann P, Langford D, Torres S, et al. Women battering in primary care practice. Fam Pract 1999; 16(4):343–352.
9. Anderson BA, Marshak HH, Hebbeler DL. Identifying intimate partner violence at entry to prenatal care: clustering routine clinical information. J Midwifery Womens Health 2002; 47(5):353–359.
10. Campbell JC, Woods AB, Laughon Chouaf K, et al. Reproductive health consequences of intimate partner violence: a nursing research review. Clin Nurs Res 2000; 9(3):217–237.
11. Harrykissoon SD, Rickert VI, Wiemann CM. Prevalence and patterns of intimate partner violence among adolescent mothers during the postpartum period. Arch Pediat Adol Med 2002; 56(4):325–330.
12. Gazmararian JA, Lazorick S, Spitz AM. Prevalence of violence against pregnant women. JAMA 1996; 275:1915–1920.
13. Sharps PW, Koziol-McLain J, Campbell, et al. Health care providers' missed opportunities for preventing femicide. Prev Med 2001; 33(5):373–380.
14. Saltzman LE, Fanslow JL, McMahon PM, et al. Intimate partner violence surveillance: uniform definitions and recommended data elements, Version 1.0. Atlanta: National Center for Injury Prevention and Control, Centers for Disease Prevention, 1999.
15. Bradley F, Smith M, Long J, et al. Reported frequency of domestic violence: cross sectional survey of women attending general practice. BMJ 2002; 324(7332):271.

16. Glass N, Dearwater S, Campbell J. Intimate partner violence screening and intervention: data from eleven Pennsylvania and California community hospital emergency departments. J Emerg Nurs 2001; 27(2):141–149.

17. Acierno RA, Resnick HS, Kilpatrick DG. Health impact of interpersonal violence: prevalence rates, case identification, and risk factors for sexual assault, physical assault, and domestic violence in men and women. Behav Med 1997; 23:53–64.

18. Bachman R, Saltzman LE. Violence against women: estimates from the redesigned Survey. Bureau of Justice Statistics Special Report: US Department of Justice NCJ-154348; 1995:1–8.

19. Plitcha S. The effects of woman abuse on health care utilization and health status: a literature review. Womens Health Issues 1992; 2:154–163.

20. Sharps PW, Campbell JC. Health consequences for victims of violence in intimate relationships. In: Arriaga XB, Oskamp S, eds. Violence in intimate relationships. Thousand Oaks: Sage; 1999:163–180.

21. Tjaden P, Thoennes N. Full report of the prevalence, incidence, and consequences of violence against women. Anonymous. Washington, DC: National Institute of Justice. (NCJ-183781); 2000.

22. Grisso JA, Wishner AR, Schwarz DF, et al. A population-based study of injuries in inner-city women. Am J Epidemiol 1991; 134:59–68.

23. Kyriacou DN, Anglin D, Taliaferro E, et al. Risk factors for injury to women from domestic violence. New Engl J Med 1999; 341(25):1892–1898.

24. Mullerman R, Lenaghan PA, Pakieser RA. Battered women: injury locations and types. Ann Emerg Med 1996; 28:486–492.

25. Vavarro FF, Lasko DL. Physical abuse as cause of injury in women: information for orthopaedic nurses. Orthop Nurs 1993; 12:37–41.

26. Zachariades N, Koumoura F, Konsolaki-Agouridake E. Facial trauma in women resulting from violence by men. J Oral Maxillofac Surg 1990; 48:1250–1253.

27. Paulozzi LJ, Saltzman LE, Thompson MP, et al. Surveillance for homicide among intimate partners: United States 1981–1998. MMWR CDC Surveill Summ 2001; 50(3):1–15.

28. Bergman B, Brismar B. A 5-year follow-up study of 117 battered women. Am J Public Health 1991; 81(11):1486–1488.

29. Eby KK, Campbell JC, Sullivan CM, et al. Health effects of experiences of sexual violence for women with abusive partners. Health Care Women Int 1995; 16:563–576.

30. Jamieson DJ, Steege JF. The association of sexual abuse with pelvic pain complaints in a primary care population. Am J Obstet Gynecol 1997; 177(6):1408–1412.

31. Leserman J, Li Z, Drossman DA, et al. Selected symptoms associated with sexual and physical abuse history among female patients with gastrointestinal disorders: the impact on subsequent health care visits. Psychol Med 1998; 28:417–425.

32. Plichta SB, Abraham C. Violence and gynecologic health in women < 50 years old. Am J Obstet Gynecol 1996; 174:903–907.

33. Schei B. Physically abusive spouse: a risk factor of pelvic inflammatory disease? Scand J Prim Health 1991; 9:41–45.

34. Schei B. Psycho-social factors in pelvic pain: a controlled study of women living in physically abusive relationships. Acta Obstet Gynecol Scand 1990; 69(1):67–71.

35. Sutherland C, Bybee D, Sullivan C. The long-term effects of battering on women's health. Womens Health 1998; 4:41–70.

36. Toomey TC, Hernandez JR, Gittleman DF, et al. Relationship of sexual and physical abuse to pain and psychological adjustment variables in chronic pelvic pain patients. Pain 1993; 53:105–109.

37. Plichta SB, Abraham C. Violence and gynecological health in women < 50 years old. Am J Obstet Gynecol 1996; 174(3):903–907.

38. Liebschutz JM, Feinman G, Sullivan L, et al. Physical and sexual abuse in women infected with the human immunodeficiency virus: increased illness and health care utilization. Arch Intern Med 2000; 160:1659–1664.

39. Coker AL, Sanderson M, Fadden MK, et al. Intimate partner violence and cervical neoplasia. J Women Health Gen-B 2000; 9(9):1015–1023.

40. Schiffman MH, Castle P. Epidemiologic studies of a necessary causal factor: human papillomavirus infection and cervical neoplasia. J Natl Cancer Inst 2003; 95:6.

41. Institute of Medicine. The hidden epidemic: confronting sexually transmitted diseases. Washington, DC: National Academy Press; 1997.

42. Turner CF, Rogers SM, Miller HG, et al. Untreated gonococcal and chlamydial infection in a probability sample of adults. JAMA 2002; 287(6):726–733.

43. Campbell JC, Soeken K. Women's responses to battering over time: an analysis of change. J Interpers Violence 1999; 14:21–40.

44. Martin SL, Matza LS, Kupper LL, et al. Domestic violence and sexually transmitted diseases: the experience of prenatal care patients. Public Health Rep 1999; 114(May/June):262–268.

45. Wingood GM, DiClemente RJ, Raj A. Adverse consequences of intimate partner abuse among women in non-urban domestic violence shelters. Am J Prev Med 2000; 19(4):270–275.

46. Champion JD, Shain RN, Piper J, et al. Sexual abuse and sexual risk behaviors of minority women with sexually transmitted diseases. West J Nurs Res 2001; 23(3):241–254.

47. Beadnell B, Baker SA, Morrison DM, et al. HIV/STD risk factors for women with violent male partners. Sex Roles 2000; 42(7/8):661–689.

48. Kalichman SC, Williams EA, Cherry C, et al. Sexual coercion, domestic violence, and negotiating condom use among low-income African American women. J Womens Health 1998; 7(3):371–378.

49. Miller M, Paone D. Social network characteristics as mediators in the relationship between sexual abuse and HIV risk. Soc Sci Med 1998; 47(6):765–777.

50. Wingood GM, DiClemente RJ. Effects of having a physically abusive partner on the condom use and sexual negotiation rates of young adult African American women. Am J Public Health 1997; 2:53–60.

51. Champion JD, Shain RN. The context of sexually transmitted disease: life histories of woman abuse. Issues Ment Health Nurs 1998; 19:463–480.

52. Davila YR, Brackley MH. Mexican and Mexican American women in a battered women's shelter: barriers to condom negotiation for HIV/AIDS prevention. Issues Ment Health Nurs 2001; 20:333–355.

53. El-Bassel N, Gilbert L, Rajah V, et al. Fear and violence: raising the HIV stakes. AIDS Educ Prev 2000.

54. Suarez-Al-Adam M, Raffaelli M, O'Leary A. Influence of abuse and partner hypermasculinity on the sexual behavior of Latinas. AIDS Educ Prev 2000; 12(3):263–274.

55. El-Bassel N, Gilbert L, Krishnan S, et al. Partner violence and sexual HIV-risk behaviors among women in an inner-city emergency department. Violence Vict 1998; 13(4):377–393.

56. Cohen M, Deamant C, Barkan S, et al. Domestic violence and childhood sexual abuse in HIV-infected women and women at risk for HIV. Am J Public Health 2000; 90(4):560–565.

57. Augenbraun M, Wilson TE, Allister L. Domestic violence reported by women attending a sexually transmitted disease clinic. Sex Transm Dis 2001; 28(3):143–147.

58. Stevens PE, Richards DJ. Narrative case analysis of HIV infection in a battered woman. Health Care Women Int 1998; 19:9–22.

59. He H, McCoy HV, Stevens SJ, et al. Violence and HIV sexual risk behaviors among female sex partners of male drug users. Women Health 1998; 27(1/2):161–175.

60. El-Bassel N, Fontdevila J, Gilbert L, et al. HIV risks of men in methadone maintenance treatment programs who abuse their intimate partners: a forgotten issue. J Subst Abuse 2001; 13:29–43.

61. McCauley J, Kern DE, Kolodner K, et al. Relation of low-severity violence to women's health. J Gen Intern Med 1998; 13:687–691.

62. Janssen PA, Holt VL, Sugg NK, et al. Intimate partner violence and adverse pregnancy outcomes: a population-based study. Am J Obstet Gynecol 2003; 188(5):1341–1347.

63. Gielen AC, O'Campo P, Faden R, et al. Interpersonal conflict and physical violence during the child-bearing years. Soc Sci Med 1994; 39:781–787.

64. Glander SS, Moore ML, Michielutte R, et al. The prevalence of domestic violence among women seeking abortion. Obstet Gynecol 1998; 91(6):1002–1006.

65. Hedin LW, Janson PO. Domestic violence during pregnancy: the prevalence of physical injuries, substance use, abortions and miscarriages. Acta Obstet Gynecol Scand 2000; 79(8):625–630.

66. Lumsden GM. Partner abuse prevalence and abortion. Can J Womens Health Care Phys Addressing Womens Health Issues 1997; 8(1):13.

67. Renker PR. Keep a blank face: I need to tell you what has been happening to me. MCN Am J Matern Child Nurs 2002; 27(2):109–116.

68. Murphy CC, Schei B, Myhr TL, et al. Abuse: a risk factor for low birth weight? A systematic review and meta-analysis. Can Med Assoc J 2001; 164(11):1567–1572.

69. McFarlane J, Campbell JC, Sharps P, et al. Abuse during pregnancy and femicide: urgent implications for women's health. Obstet Gynecol 2002; 100(1):27–36.

70. McFarlane J, Soeken K. Weight change of infants age birth to 12 months born to abused women. Pediatr Nurs 1999; 25(1):19–23.

71. Campbell JC, Lewandowski LA. Mental and physical health effects of intimate partner violence on women and children. Psychiatr Clin N Am 1997; 20(2):353–373.

72. Wisner CL, Gilmer TP, Saltzman LE, et al. Intimate partner violence against women: do victims cost health plans more? J Fam Practice 1999; 48(6):439–443.

73. Plitcha S. The effects of woman abuse on health care utilization and health status. Womens Health Issues 1992; 2(3):154–163.

74. Coker AL, Watkins KW, Smith PH, et al. Social support reduces the impact of partner violence on health: application of structural equation models. Prev Med 2003; 37:259–267.

75. Nurius PS, Macy RJ, Bhuyan R, et al. Contextualizing depression and physical functioning in battered women. J Interpers Violence 2003; 18(12):1411–1431.

76. Zink T, Sill M. Intimate partner violence and job stability. J Am Med Womens Assoc 2004; 59(1):32–35.

77. Gerlock AA. Health impact of domestic violence. Issues Ment Health Nurs 1999; 20:373–385.

78. Gleason WJ. Mental disorders in battered women: an empirical study. Violence Vict 1993; 8(1):53–68.

79. Roberts GL, Williams GM, Lawrence JM, et al. How does domestic violence affect women's mental health? Women Health 1998; 28(1):117–129.

80. West CG, Fernandez A, Hillard JR, et al. Psychiatric disorders of abused women at a shelter. Psychiatr Q 1990; 61(4):295–301.

81. Golding JM. Intimate partner violence as a risk factor for mental disorders: a meta-analysis. J Fam Violence 1999; 14(2):99–132.

82. Hegarty K, Gunn J, Chondros P, et al. Association between depression and abuse by partners of women attending general practice: descriptive, cross sectional survey. Brit Med J 2004; 328:621–624.

83. Coid J, Petrukevitch A, Chung W, et al. Abusive experiences and psychiatric comorbidity in women primary care attenders. Br J Psychiatry 2003; 183:332–9.

84. Campbell JC, Kub J, Belknap RA, et al. Predictors of depression in battered women. Violence Against Women 1997; 3:271–293.

85. Cascardi M, O'Leary KD, Schlee KA. Co-occurrence and correlates of posttraumatic stress disorder and major depression in physically abused women. J Fam Violence 1999; 14:227–250.

86. Astin MC, Lawrence KJ, Foy DW. Posttraumatic stress disorder among battered women: risk and resiliency factors. Violence Vict 1993; 8(1):17–28.

87. Astin MC, Ogland-Hand SM, Coleman EM, et al. Posttraumatic stress disorder and childhood abuse in battered women: comparisons with maritally distressed women. J Consult Clin Psych 1995; 63(2):308–312.

88. Houskamp B, Foy DW. The assessment of posttraumatic stress disorder in battered women. J Interpers Violence 1991; 6(3):367–375.

89. Vitanza S, Vogel LCM, Marshall LL. (1995). Distress and symptoms of posttraumatic stress disorder in abused women. Violence Vict 1995; 10(1):23–34.

90. Woods SJ. Prevalence and patterns of posttraumatic stress disorder in abused and postabused women. Issues Ment Health Nurs 2000; 21(3):309–324.

91. Breslau N, Kessler RC, Chilcoat HD, et al. Trauma and posttraumatic stress disorder in the community. Arch Gen Psychiatry 1998; 55:626–632.

92. Kessler RC, Sonnega A, Bromet E, et al. Posttraumatic stress disorder in the National Comorbidity Survey. Arch Gen Psychiatry 1995; 52:1048–1060.

93. Stein MB, Kennedy C. Major depressive and post-traumatic stress disorder comorbidity in female victims of intimate partner violence. J Affect Disorders 2001; 66(2–3):133–138.

94. O'Campo P, Kub J, Woods A, et al. Depression, PTSD and comorbidity related to intimate partner violence in civilian and military women. Unpublished manuscript.

95. Silverman JG, Raj A, Mucci LA, et al. Dating violence against adolescent girls and associated substance use, unhealthy weight control, sexual risk behavior, pregnancy, and suicidality. JAMA 2001; 286(5):572–579.

96. Hirschfeld RMA. The comorbidity of major depression and anxiety disorders: recognition and management in primary care. Prim Care Companion J Clin Psychiatry 2001; 3:244–254.

97. Ballenger JC, Davidson JRT, Lecrubier Y, et al. Consensus statement on posttraumatic stress disorder from the International Consensus Group on Depression and Anxiety. J Clin Psychiatry 2000; 61(Suppl. 5):60–66.

98. Logan T, Walker R, Cole J, et al. Victimization and substance abuse. Rev Gen Psychol (in press).

99. Kilpatrick DG, Acierno R, Resick HS, et al. A two-year longitudinal analysis of the relationships between violent assault and substance use in women. J Consult Clin Psych 1997; 65:834–847.

100. El-Bassel N, Gilbert L, Krishnan S, et al. Partner violence and sexual HIV-risk behaviors among women in an inner-city emergency department. Violence Vict 1998; 13(4):377–393.

101. Kalichman SC, Williams EA, Cherry C, et al. Sexual coercion, domestic violence, and negotiating condom use among low-income African American women. J Women Health 1998; 7(3):371–378.

102. Coker AL, Smith PH, Bethea L, et al. Physical health consequences of physical and psychological intimate partner violence. Arch Fam Med 2000; 9(5):451–457.

103. Wilson-Cohn C, Strauss SM, Falkin GP. The relationship between partner abuse and substance use among women mandated to drug treatment. J Fam Violence 2002; 17(1):91–105.

104. Miller BA. Partner violence experiences and women's drug use: exploring the connections. In: Galante M, ed. Recent developments in alcoholism, Vol. 13: Alcoholism and violence. New York: Plenum Press; 1997:407–416.

105. Letourneau EJ, Holmes M, Chasedunn-Roark J. Gynecological health consequences to victims of interpersonal violence. Womens Health Issues 1999; 9(2):115–120.

106. Wingood GM, DiClemente RJ, Raj A. Adverse consequences of intimate partner abuse among women in non-urban domestic violence shelters. Am J Prev Med 2000; 19(4):270–275.

107. Grant EG, Campbell JC. Abuse, drugs, and crime: pathways to a vicious cycle. J Add Nurs 1998; 10(1):15–27.

108. Dembo D, Dertke M, LaVoie L, et al. Physical abuse, sexual victimization, and illicit drug use: a structural analysis among high risk adolescents. J Adolescence 1987; 19:13–33.

109. Burnam MA, Stein JA, Golding JM, et al. Sexual assault and mental disorders in a community population. J Consult Clin Psych 1988; 56(6):843–850.

110. Schuck AM, Widom CS. Childhood victimization and alcohol symptoms in females: causal inferences and hypothesized mediators. Child Abuse Neglect 2001; 25(8):1069–1092.

111. Epstein JN, Saunders BE, Kilpatrick DG, et al. PTSD as a mediator between childhood rape and alcohol use in adult women. Child Abuse Neglect 1998; 22(3):223–234.

112. Jacobsen LK, Southwick SM, Kosten TR. Substance use disorders in patients with posttraumatic stress disorder: a review of the literature. Am J Psychol 2001; 158(8):1184–1190.

113. Chilcoat HD, Breslau N. Posttraumatic stress disorder and drug disorders: testing causal pathways. Arch Gen Psychiatry 1998; 55:913–917.

114. Breslau N, Davis GC, Peterson EL, et al. Psychiatric sequelae of stress disorder in women. Arch Gen Psychiatry 1997; 54:81–87.

115. Kessler RC, McGonagle KA, Zhao S, et al. Lifetime and 12-month prevalence of DSM-III-R psychiatric disorders in the United States: results from the National Comorbidity Survey. Arch Gen Psychiatry 1994; 51(1):8–19.

116. Widom CS, Weiler BL, Cottler LB. Childhood victimization and drug abuse: a comparison of prospective and retrospective findings. J Consult Clin Psychol 1999; 67(6):867–880.

117. MacMillan HL, Fleming JE, Streiner DL, et al. Childhood abuse and lifetime psychopathology in a community sample. Am J Psychol 2001; 158(11):1878–1883.

118. Kessler RC, Sonnega A, Bromet E, et al. Posttraumatic stress disorder in the National Comorbidity Survey. Arch Gen Psychiatry 1995; 52:1048–1060.

119. Diaz-Olavarrieta C, Campbell JC, Garcia de la Cadena C, et al. Domestic violence against patients with chronic neurologic disorders. Arch Neurol 1999; 56:681–685.

120. Irwin C, Falsetti SA, Lydiard RB, et al. Comorbidity of posttraumatic stress disorder and irritable bowel syndrome. J Clin Psychiatry 1996; 57(12):576–578.

121. Talley N, Fett SL, Zinsmeister AR. Self-reported abuse and gastrointestinal disease in outpatients: association with irritable bowel-type symptoms. Am J Gastroenterol 1995; 90(3):366–371.

122. Talley N, Fett SL, Zinsmeister AR, et al. Gastrointestinal tract symptoms and self-reported abuse: a population-based study. Gastroenterology 1994; 107:1040–1049.

123. Rabin BS. Stress, immune function, and health: the connection. New York: John Wiley; 1999.

124. Rice VH, ed. Handbook of stress, coping, and health: implications for nursing research, theory, and practice. Thousand Oaks, CA: Sage; 2000.

125. Constantino RE, Sekula LK, Rabin B, et al. Negative life experiences, depression, and immune function in abused and nonabused women. Biol Res Nurs 2000; 1(3):190–198.

126. Wilson SN, van der Kolk B, Burbridge J, et al. Phenotype of blood lymphocytes in PTSD suggests chronic immune activation. Psychosomatics 1999; 40(3):222–225.

127. Campbell JC, Ryan H, Campbell DW, et al. Physical and nonphysical abuse and other risk factors for low birthweight among term and preterm babies: a multiethnic case control study. Am J Epidemiol 1999; 150:714–726.

128. McFarlane J, Parker B, Soeken K. Abuse during pregnancy: associations with maternal health and infant birth weight. Nur Res 1996; 45:37–42.

Chapter 4

Educating health professionals: changing attitudes and overcoming barriers

Carole Warshaw, Angela Taft, and Heather McCosker-Howard

I don't want health professionals to solve it. I want them to be able to intervene. That means listen, believe, help women with resources. You know, be willing to be with them where they are at, whatever their choices turn out to be.

General practitioner trainer about working with women survivors of IPA

CHAPTER CONTENTS

INTRODUCTION

Addressing intimate partner abuse (IPA) presents unique challenges for individual practitioners and for the institutions that shape health care education and practice. In addition to the need for acquiring new knowledge and skills, health professionals are faced with the task of confronting the feelings and social beliefs that shape their responses to patients. They also need to develop new frameworks for understanding complex social issues and to generate collaborative models for working in multidisciplinary teams and in partnership with community advocacy groups.

Educators, in turn, must be able to provide training experiences that foster the development of those understandings and skills; institutional structures that support their integration into routine practice; and faculty who model non-abusive behaviour in all aspects of training and clinical care.[1-2]

Collaboration between health care providers and advocates for women experiencing partner abuse has generated a model based on principles of prevention, safety, empowerment, advocacy, accountability, and social change.[3-5] Translating these principles into new standards of care, however, will require a paradigm shift for many health professionals as well as changes in teaching strategies and in the health care system itself.[5, 6] Identifying and overcoming the barriers encountered by health professionals as they attempt to incorporate public health and advocacy-based concepts provides an opportunity to rethink our philosophies and methods of professional training. It also provides the opportunity to develop more sophisticated models for understanding the problems faced by patients and to examine how the structure of clinical education affects the ability of health professionals to provide optimal care.[1] Recent studies evaluating outcomes of training on IPA underscore these challenges and highlight the difficulties providers have integrating knowledge about IPA into practice unless these broader issues are addressed.[7-9]

This chapter offers suggestions for changes in health professional education that will assist practitioners to address the complex issues they face in responding to IPA and to incorporate appropriate identification and intervention for IPA into the core of their clinical work. The chapter also offers suggestions for changes in the structure and content of professional education as part of generating a health care system response to preventing IPA and its long-term consequences. These suggestions apply to undergraduate and postgraduate clinical training as well as to practising health professionals. We acknowledge that abuse occurs in same-sex relationships (see Chapter 13), but we will refer to victim/survivors as 'she' and perpetrators as 'he' for reasons stated in the Preface of this book.

Limits of traditional models

In order to understand the issues raised by IPA, health professionals must first become familiar with the prevalence, impact, dynamics, and social underpinnings of abuse. However, developing curricula that include this type of information will require a more comprehensive framework than that offered by traditional biomedical approaches. A key limitation of these models centres on the difficulty of incorporating complex social issues into a conceptual framework designed primarily to address medical problems – a framework that too often masks important underlying concerns. Health professionals are reluctant to delve beyond the obvious for a variety of reasons.[10–13] Until recently, Western-trained health professionals were educated to treat physical injuries without regard to underlying cause, and remained relatively unaware of the impact of IPA on patients' health and well-being. When we treat only the physical or mental health symptoms that result from IPA, without a clear awareness of the context in which they occur, we are less prepared to understand and respond to the range of issues patients themselves must confront.[14–16]

For example, during training sessions health professionals often describe their inability to understand why a woman will not 'admit' she is being abused when it seems so obvious to the practitioner, or why she will not leave an abusive partner when she is clearly in danger. A framework that recognizes the psychological entrapment from which a woman must extricate herself, the ways that entrapment is reinforced by the threats she may face if she decides to disclose or leave, and a social context in which options for living safely and independently may be limited, can help clinicians respond more empathically and effectively.[16]

Thus, what appears to the clinician to be a constellation of symptoms or disorders may reflect a response, not just to the physical or psychic trauma of chronic abuse and violence, but also to the social realities of ongoing isolation and danger. A purely clinical focus also fails to acknowledge the role of practitioner–patient interactions in reinforcing or transforming the experience of abuse. When health professionals do not ask about abuse or make it safe for patients to respond, they inadvertently contribute to the despair a survivor may feel, the prolongation of her symptoms, and her continued exposure to danger.[3,5] Without a more comprehensive framework – one that views social issues as central to patients' health and well-being – asking about abuse becomes yet another add-on, rather than an integral part of clinical routines.

TEACHING MORE COMPLEX MODELS

Public health and advocacy models add important contextual dimensions that help broaden perspective, deepen understanding, and expand the scope of potential interventions.[17] Understanding IPA requires an ability to conceptualize the forces that sustain a perpetrator's motivation and ability to abuse or control a partner; the contextual factors that mediate patients' experiences of abuse and shape their options; and the individual and systemic factors that determine providers' responses to this issue.[18,19] Although research has not systematically assessed the effects of more subtle forms of social and cultural victimization, many authors describe the importance of understanding how discrimination due to gender, race, ethnicity, sexual orientation, disability, and socioeconomic status also affect an individual's experience of abuse.[16,20]

By expanding the traditional 'pathology-in-the-patient' model to include social context, the 'problem' or 'pathology' can be redefined as the perpetrator's abusive behavior; societal beliefs that tolerate or condone the abuse; and the social, cultural, and political–economic structures that sustain, support, and mediate its impact. Interventions derived from such a model would address women's social as well as physical and psychological realities, and provide more realistic opportunities for prevention. It is also important for practitioners to be aware that while some of the problems faced by survivors of IPA can be addressed through medical or mental health interventions, others are best addressed through advocacy and social change.

As health professionals become more skilled at recognizing the sequelae of abuse and at addressing the immediate safety needs of victims, they may be faced with the frustrations of working within increasingly rigid time constraints, the realities of limited community resources, and an inadequate criminal justice response[12,21] (e.g. policies and laws such as mandatory reporting of IPA that can endanger women, or work against women's health needs – see Chapter 10). Knowledge of the legal system, community resources, and strategies to protect women's safety, as well as steps practitioners can take to influence policies that affect their patients' health and well-being, are also essential components of a framework for teaching about IPA.

THE SOCIAL CONSTRUCTION OF ABUSE AND CLINICAL INSTITUTIONS

Analysing the social construction of IPA provides another vehicle for understanding how the personal, social, and political can intersect to sustain the dynamics of abuse. For example, individual perpetrators have not only the psychological need but also the social permission to terrorize and control their partners. To a large extent, such psychological need is constructed within a context where the expression of needs often takes highly gendered forms.[22,23] Understanding these dynamics requires shifting from a strictly clinical perspective to one that recognizes the relationship between clinical problems, cultural values, gender, and social institutions.[24–26] While these power dynamics are largely organized along gender lines, particularly in heterosexual partner abuse, physical capacity, emotional vulnerability, age, stigma, and social status can also play significant roles in IPA.

Understanding IPA can also lead to greater comprehension of other types of abuse in which social norms intersect with individual needs to create abusive dynamics. Professional status provides one potential vehicle for the abuse of power. While power differentials in any work or educational environment can create opportunities for abuse, there are aspects of professional socialization that can also contribute to these dynamics, particularly in high-stress settings where detachment and control are privileged over attention to context and feelings. If interpersonal or psychosocial aspects of care are not valued or reimbursed, practitioners are less likely to develop or utilize their capacities to attend to these issues. And, if health professionals learn to tolerate abusive behaviour when it occurs in their own training or work environments, they may find it more difficult to respond appropriately to patients who are being abused.[27,28]

A model that is sufficiently complex and dynamic to address the societal contexts that produce and shape the experience of abuse must address the conditions that shape clinicians' interactions with victimized and abusive patients. It must also acknowledge the need to transform conditions that limit health professionals' abilities to respond.[6]

Providing this kind of framework and creating supportive training environments are necessary for health professionals to address the complicated issues raised in integrating information about IPA. If we can begin to understand what sustains and transforms abusive power dynamics in both individual and institutional forms, we can perhaps begin to develop a template for changing those dynamics within our own institutions, communities, and lives. Such wide-ranging institutional and curricular reform requires educational leadership, mutual respect, and collaboration.

CORE CURRICULAR PRINCIPLES, COMPETENCIES, AND EDUCATIONAL STRATEGIES FOR TEACHING ABOUT IPA

Since the 1990s, a number of tertiary institutions and advocacy groups have begun to develop and test core curricular principles and competencies as well as a range of educational strategies to help produce more appropriate and effective health professional responses to patients experiencing IPA.[4,29–32] These activities have mainly focused on the health professionals' role in working with victims – in part because the impetus for addressing IPA in health care settings came from victim advocates and survivors who could provide clear guidance on what would and would not be helpful and safe.

Recent public health understandings of prevention, early intervention, and the impact of IPA on children require additional changes in health professional curricula to include education about the clinician's role in identifying and treating patients who are abusers, working with couples when abuse may be a concern, and providing interventions for children exposed to IPA.[33–39] For example, clinicians need to be aware of the dangers of couples' therapy when there is ongoing violence and the importance of working with children in ways that support the non-abusive parent. They also need a clear understanding of abusive dynamics and how to intervene safely with patients who are abusing their partners[40–42] (see Chapter 9). Some of these issues are already being incorporated into longer preclinical courses on family violence and into paediatric and mental health curricula.[43–45]

Increasingly, studies evaluating the effects of training on clinician response to IPA have emphasized the need to establish core competencies for health professionals, to institute educational policy reforms and institutional supports, and to build partnerships with community advocacy groups.[46–51] While there are a number of models for training health professionals about IPA, recommended education and practice reforms generally reflect the following core principles:[46]

- The immediate and long-term safety of the patient is the first guiding principle of assessment and intervention for IPA.
- Routine inquiry conducted in a confidential, non-judgmental, and compassionate manner is an essential skill that needs to become a part of routine care.

- Understanding the dynamics of abuse, respecting survivors' choices, and holding perpetrators accountable for their abusive behaviour are critical to appropriate intervention.
- Education should include information on the legal protections available for adult and child victims of abuse as well as the legal and reporting requirements for health care providers and institutions in relation to IPA (see Chapter 10).
- Professionals need to understand the rationale and develop the skills to work effectively as part of a multidisciplinary team. This includes working in collaboration with advocacy groups and developing ways to link survivors to community resources.
- Health professionals also need to develop an awareness of their own responses and behaviour and how these can affect clinical care.
- Interventions and responses should reflect an understanding of the cultural background, needs, and preferences of patients being served.
- Health professionals can play a role in preventing abuse and its consequences by engaging in individual and systems advocacy; participating in broader community responses to IPA; and working to change social norms that foster abuse and violence.

Curriculum content also varies across settings, although core elements are relatively consistent as well (i.e. overview of problem, identification, assessment, basic intervention, documentation, and referral). Curricular learning objectives and skill-based competencies should include the following:

- Problem awareness, (prevalence, impact, presentations).
- Dynamics of IPA and social context.
- IPA across diverse communities.
- Issues of safety, privacy, confidentiality, validation, and empowerment.
- Identification, assessment, and diagnosis.
- Intervention and treatment (including addressing safety, providing information, discussing options).
- Documentation.
- Legal protections and responses.
- Community resources and referrals.
- Additional clinical issues (e.g. parenting in the context of IPA; addressing lifetime trauma; mental health; and substance abuse in the context of IPA).
- Controversial issues (e.g. screening male patients for victimization and perpetration; when and how to address battering).
- Provider issues, responses, and concerns.
- Prevention, collaboration, advocacy, and social change.

Differences in educational content and teaching strategies often reflect the amount of time a programme or institution is willing to invest in these activities. This can range from a less-than-an-hour in-service to a full semester course. Training conducted in clinical settings tends to be shorter and more focused on practical knowledge and skills. Lack of attention to provider issues, lack of opportunities to solidify new skills, lack of institutional reinforcement, and lack of community collaboration can all have an impact on their effectiveness.

For example, despite the curricular principles listed above, a recent US national evaluation of nurse practitioner training found that legal issues and the safety of survivors and children were least likely to be taught.[7] Another study, evaluating a four-week medical student training programme on IPA found that differences in learning outcomes between groups of students depended on tutors' own attitudes and levels of preparedness.[47] They also found the programme to be more successful in creating student motivation to identify IPA than in generating student confidence in their ability to inquire and respond. Students were also keen to intervene, but without adequate sensitivity to women's ability to be able to act. While training on recognition and intervention for IPA does increase the likelihood that health professionals will identify and respond appropriately to survivors of domestic abuse, overall, these models have been more effective at improving knowledge and confidence than at changing actual practice.[3–5,51] Again, this points to the need for both curricular and institutional changes that address the obstacles practitioners face in responding to IPA.

Creating a supportive environment for learning

Because interpersonal skills are such an important component of responding to IPA, curricula need to include interactive teaching activities as well. For example, standard didactic formats provide neither sufficient opportunity to address the attitudes and feelings that may affect a clinician's ability to provide appropriate care, nor sufficient room to acquire the skills necessary for an optimal response. And, although the majority of health professionals may be aware that IPA is a significant social and health problem, there are clearly barriers that prevent or minimize their response to patients experiencing IPA (see Chapter 5). Therefore, it is vital for educators to create learning environments that offer the emotional safety to explore cultural and personal responses to abuse and opportunities to discuss individual, professional, and institutional concerns. While one-time trainings may raise awareness, ongoing feedback and support are necessary to develop and sustain provider response.

Feelings that arise in talking to patients about abuse

Health professionals have to be able to acknowledge their own emotional responses to hearing about abuse, be able to tolerate what they hear, and remain professional yet available to their patients. Clinical education does not always address the psychological impact of hearing patients discuss painful situations, particularly ones the clinician is unable to fix or in which a patient's choices conflict with those of the clinician. The feelings of helplessness that arise when we see someone living with pain or fear that we cannot make go away can be difficult to tolerate. Moreover, many health professionals will have experienced abuse in their own families or relationships and may find it hard to address such issues and the feelings evoked by them, unless there is a safe atmosphere in which they can do so. For those for whom this experience comes too close to home, it may be even more difficult to risk having painful feelings evoked while trying to function in a professional capacity.[2] Acknowledging the likelihood of personal experience of IPA and offering recognition and support is often a useful and important starting point.

Professionals also have to deal with the feelings that arise when faced with expectations of functioning competently in areas where they do not yet have the skill or expertise. When we ask health professionals to screen for IPA, it is not the same as screening for heart disease or colon cancer. Clinicians report being afraid of 'opening Pandora's Box', and perhaps more importantly, of not knowing what to do or how to handle what they may hear.[52]

Creating space for trainees to practice skills, explore possible responses, and discuss challenging clinical interactions without fear of embarrassment is another way to assist practitioners to develop their capacities to respond to IPA. Not only do trainees have to attend to patients' feelings at the same time that they may be struggling with their own; they are also faced with asking a host of new questions, offering unfamiliar interventions, and trying to be helpful in situations that are beyond the purview of traditional clinical care. Having access to experienced clinicians or faculty who can model ways to raise an issue or phrase a question, or gently push them to articulate what is behind their discomfort and their expectations for themselves and their patients, also helps trainees develop and solidify new skills.

When health professionals – particularly those still in training – begin to feel comfortable with the range of feelings that can be evoked through clinical encounters, they feel less afraid to listen to their patients, and less frustrated when they are not able to make things better or to fix a situation that is not in their control.[40] These skills may also be new to experienced practitioners who have not focused on these kinds of issues in their clinical work.

ADDITIONAL TEACHING STRATEGIES

In addition to providing core information on IPA and creating safe environments for trainees to understand their own responses, there are a number of experiential learning activities that can help clinicians to broaden their perspectives and integrate their new knowledge and skills.

Learning from survivors

Listening to women who have survived IPA talk about their lives, particularly in interactive formats, helps health professionals to understand the experience of becoming trapped in an abusive relationship and how randomly that can occur. They hear the difficult choices and obstacles women face in trying to end the violence in their lives, and the kinds of interventions they have found most helpful. They come away with a new level of respect for the dignity and strength that so many women exhibit in the face of terrible situations.[40]

Women who have experienced abuse can be found through domestic violence community services and should be paid and supported to participate in training sessions.[42] In the absence of women who are available to assist

> **Box 4.1   A practical exercise for health professionals to learn more about their own responses**[48]
>
> Trainees break into pairs or triads, and each spends five or ten minutes describing an experience in which he or she has felt victimized in some way. They are instructed to talk about what it felt like when this was happening, notice what feelings arise as they are talking, indicate what responses from their partners make them want to be more open, and describe which responses make them want to retreat. The third person plays the role of observer to provide additional feedback about non-verbal aspects of the interaction. Participants are often surprised by how vivid their feelings are, even when they are describing seemingly minor events that may have happened many years before. They also become exquisitely aware of how difficult it can be to talk about situations that evoke intense feelings, particularly if they are ones of vulnerability or shame. When they play the role of 'listener' they learn how hard it is to sit with someone else's pain, and how much more difficult it is to feel compassion when one also feels compelled to 'do something', especially when one does not know what to do. In addition, they can tell each other what it felt like when the other responded or did not respond in particular ways.

there are a variety of excellent DVDs and videotapes of survivors talking about their experiences of abuse that can be substituted.[43] Where possible, accounts from men who have stopped abusing partners are also useful in motivating professionals to learn more about working effectively with patients who abuse their partners. Again, addressing IPA with patients who are perpetrators is more complicated and potentially more endangering than working with survivors and should be undertaken only with adequate training and supervision[56] (see Chapter 9).

Simulated patients

When learners require opportunities to explore attitudes and to practise skills of inquiry and history taking, simulated patients,[57,58] problem-based cases and role playing can be helpful tools.[29] Simulated patients are non-clinicians (usually actors) who have been trained to play the role of a patient to help students develop clinical skills. Simulated patients are also useful in effectively evaluating whether skills have been sufficiently developed.[50] In addition, feedback from simulated patients can be critical to help students develop awareness of their communication skills, especially their ability to listen, empathize, and respond in empowering versus disempowering ways.

Preventing retraumatization: learning from empowerment models

Relational skill-building activities can also help practitioners become more aware of the impact they have on patients, and sensitize them to the ways in which clinical interactions can be potentially retraumatizing to survivors of abuse.[5,59] For example, Rieker and Carmen eloquently describe the denial and 'disconfirmation' of experience perpetuated by the abuser and often internalized by the victim that can be paralleled by invalidating, blaming, or pathologizing responses from the health care system itself, and from providers who have learned to protect themselves from uncomfortable feelings at the expense of their own awareness. If a health professional is unable to recognize and validate patients' experiences of abuse or the traumatic contexts in which their symptoms developed, revictimization can take place.[59]

In addition, the pressure under current practice arrangements to make rapid assessments, diagnoses, and treatment recommendations can push clinicians into a mode of taking charge and maintaining control of clinical encounters.[12,21,] For someone whose life is controlled and dominated by another person, the subtly disempowering quality of many clinical interactions can reinforce the idea that this is what is to be expected and adapted to in order to survive. How one asks questions and the safety of the setting in which questions are asked also have a tremendous impact on the messages that are received by patients as well as the information that is obtained.[15,61,62] The nature of the clinical interaction itself can either provide relief and hope or increase despair and entrapment.[63–65]

For someone who has been abused, experiencing equality, safety, mutuality, and empowerment are essential to the process of healing and reclaiming one's sense of self and place in the world. In situations when the harm to one's self is inflicted through a relationship, it is often necessary for the 'undoing' and rebuilding to take place through other relationships. The quality of those relationships are central to the healing process.

One of the greatest challenges raised by this issue is teaching health professionals to relate in ways that are truly empowering, particularly in settings where these qualities are not rewarded or valued. In order to accomplish this goal, health professionals need times during their training when they can listen to survivors without bearing responsibility for outcomes and thus feel freer to attend to their own internal responses.[26,27] It is also helpful to hear – from faculty and from survivors – how important it is just to be listened to and understood. Again, role plays, modelling by educators and advocates, simulated patients, video and in-person observation, and conversations with survivors, are all useful tools for helping health professionals learn to interact in ways that are both respectful and empowering. Advocacy perspectives provide a model for facilitating rather than directing change.

The importance of educators modelling non–abusive behaviours

In order for clinicians to learn to create empowering interactions with patients, however, they must have some experience of being responded to respectfully and empathically themselves. Educators must be aware of the importance of modelling these types of interactions not only with patients but also with colleagues and trainees. In addition, health care institutions and training programmes must provide clear messages that abuse, discrimination, and harassment will not be tolerated and develop policies and programmes to address these issues when they arise.

Modelling respectful community collaboration

Health professionals may be offered a view of their potential support and role in the wider community through site visits to community agencies such as domestic violence agencies, shelters, and courts; also by including staff from perpetrators' programmes, legal advocacy projects, and programmes that link child protective and domestic violence services as trainers. These activities can provide clinicians with a broader perspective on what survivors deal with as they engage in what is often a slow and dangerous process and enable them to be more supportive and helpful. For example, learning to help an abused woman assess her level of danger and options for safety requires a tolerance for facing the terror and danger with her, while understanding the limits of the systems designed to protect her. This process can be facilitated by creating opportunities for health professionals to work collaboratively with community programmes committed to ending IPA, and to learn from those with more expertise in these areas. This type of strategy has been successfully modelled in a number of programmes including a community partnership designed to prepare nursing students to respond to domestic violence.[66]

Clearly, clinicians working alone cannot meet all the needs of patients who are abused, nor can they realistically prevent IPA. Working in multi-disciplinary teams enriches learning and provides better coordination of services for survivors of IPA. It provides a support network for health professionals who are helping patients deal with very complicated situations – situations that require the input of a more diverse group of providers. For example, knowing what is likely to happen when a woman goes to court or calls the police in a given community, what happens when referrals are made to a particular perpetrators' programme, or what resources are available when both the children and the mother are being abused, helps practitioners reframe their notions of success and understand their roles within a larger community response.

Given the increasing time constraints placed upon clinicians in most practice settings, balance can be difficult to negotiate. Many harbour a strong sense of responsibility and feel conflict about raising personal issues when they do not feel they have the time to respond, or the expertise and resources to resolve the 'problem'. Health professionals feel more comfortable asking about abuse if they know a legal advocate to call, or a mental health provider who is skilled at dealing with trauma, or a substance-abuse programme that is sensitive to IPA. It also helps to learn that most women want to be asked about abuse, providing it is in a caring, non-judgemental way;[15] that offering validation, respect, and concern are themselves powerful interventions; and that while assessing immediate safety is critical, more in-depth interventions can be provided by an advocate or social worker, if clinicians are unable to do this themselves.

Becoming part of a community-wide effort to prevent abuse and its consequences can also help motivate health professionals to engage in thinking critically about social policy and community change.[67–70]

Potential for vicarious traumatization of health professionals

Even experienced health professionals may be confronted with addressing the traumatic impact of IPA without having the support or skills to do so. Again, this is doubly problematic when coupled with the constraints of working in practice settings that limit one's ability to take time with patients and make appropriate referrals for psychological interventions. Mental health practitioners and advocates who work extensively with trauma survivors are generally more attuned to the impact this work has on providers and to the need for ongoing support.

The concept of vicarious traumatization refers to the indirect traumatization one may experience in bearing witness to the traumatic experiences of others.[71,72] Health professionals who have experienced some form of abuse or violence themselves run the additional risk of being retraumatized in ways that affect not only them but also their abilities to remain open to their patients' experiences.[73]

Strategies for addressing vicarious traumatization include a combination of peer support and supervision that offers ongoing opportunities for trainees to discuss these issues as they arise. Peer support groups help students express and process complicated feelings that are evoked during the course of their training around a range of difficult issues, including abuse. They can provide the emotional safety to explore feelings that are difficult to face in isolation, expand one's range of options for dealing with similar experiences, and create a sense of empowerment to handle situations that feel too overwhelming to deal with alone.

For practising health professionals, working in multidisciplinary teams can serve some of these functions by providing support and perspective, reducing isolation, and helping us to feel part of a larger community response. Additional strategies such as talking with trusted colleagues, finding good supervision, obtaining outside consultation, maintaining close relationships with friends and family, and engaging in other meaningful activities, can help practitioners recognize and attend to the deeper feelings that may be evoked by this work. Maintaining a balance between professional responsibilities and personal lives, and recognizing the importance of taking care of oneself if one wants to sustain the ability to take care of others, can also mitigate the effects of vicarious traumatization.

ADDRESSING STRUCTURAL BARRIERS: CREATING INSTITUTIONAL AND SYSTEM CHANGE

In order for health professionals to develop and sustain appropriate responses to IPA, they must have the support of the institutions in which they practise. Addressing this issue requires changes in the nature of health education and in the culture of health institutions.[28] Creating practice environments and policies that support health professionals' efforts to address complex issues and that reimburse the more time-consuming tasks of listening and advocating for change are important components of institutionalizing effective responses to IPA.

Health professionals can also play an important role in helping refocus clinical, research, and training priorities, and making sure that health care organizations, legislators, and policy makers begin to recognize that the long-term consequences of non-intervention far exceed the costs of intervention and prevention.[36,74] Finally, there are a number of significant roles health professionals can play in improving health care system capacity to address IPA, such as ensuring that information about IPA is integrated into curricula, training programmes, and intake consultations, and implementing procedures that support inquiry, appropriate assessment, documentation, intervention, and referral. They can develop liaisons between health care providers and domestic violence advocacy groups in the community, and work to ensure reimbursement for services needed by patients who are being abused by an intimate partner.

CONCLUSION

Learning about IPA raises complex issues for health professionals. In order for them to be able to address these issues educators must create supportive training environments. This will help them develop the skills and capacities to respond effectively to patients who have been abused. Expanding traditional health paradigms to develop a framework of sufficient breadth and complexity to address the multiple dimensions of abuse can begin to lay the groundwork for such a process. In addition, health professionals need to be encouraged to develop awareness of the larger social forces that affect both individual and public health and to recognize their potential roles as community members in reducing IPA. An important part of these roles is working collaboratively in multidisciplinary community partnerships.

Some of the above suggestions for changes in the structure of professional education are first steps in the process of creating a health care system contribution to reducing and preventing IPA. One way to do this is by creating a model for fostering non-abusive relationships at both individual and institutional levels within the health care system, thus developing a paradigm for transforming conditions that produce and sustain abuse.

A critical role for educators is the regular and rigorous evaluation of training programmes to ensure that learning objectives and strategies are effective. Regular and sustained process evaluation will ensure that IPA education and training programmes continue to improve and strengthen in their effectiveness.

REFERENCES

1. Warshaw C. Limitations of the medical model in the care of battered women. Gender Soc 1989; 3:506–517.
2. Warshaw C. Domestic violence: challenges to medical practice. J Women Health 1993; 2:73–80.
3. Sassetti M. Domestic violence. Prim Care 1993; 20(2):289–305.
4. Brandt Jr EN. Curricular principles for health professions education about family violence. Acad Med 1997; 72(Jan Suppl. 1): S51–58.
5. Gondolf EW. Assessing woman battering in mental health services. Thousand Oaks, CA: Sage; 1998.

6. Warshaw C. Domestic violence: changing theory, changing practice. J Am Med Womens Assoc 1996; 51(3):87–91.

7. Hinderliter D, Doughty AS, Delaney K, et al. The effect of intimate partner violence education on nurse practitioners' feelings of competence and ability to screen patients. J Nurs Educ 2003; 42(10):449–454.

8. Jonassen JA, Mazor KM. Identification of physician and patient attributes that influence the likelihood of screening for intimate partner violence. Acad Med 2003; 78(10 Suppl. l): S20–23.

9. Sitterding HAT, Adera T, Shield-Fobbs E. Spouse/partner violence education as a predictor of screening practices among physicians. J Contin Educ Health Prof 2003; 23(1):54–63.

10. Mezey G, Bacchus L, Haworth A, et al. Midwives' perceptions and experience of routine enquiry for domestic violence. Brit J Obstet Gynaec 2003; 110:744–752.

11. Woodtli MA. Nurses' attitudes towards survivors and perpetrators of domestic violence. J Holistic Nurs 2001; 19(4):340–359.

12. Elliott L, Nerney M, Jones T, et al. Barriers to screening for domestic violence. J Int Med 2002; 17:112–116.

13. Taket A, Nurse J, Smith K, et al. Routinely asking women about domestic violence in health settings. BMJ 2003; 327:673–676.

14. Sharps PW, Koziol-McLain J, Campbell JC, et al. Health care providers' missed opportunities for preventing femicide. Prev Med 2001; 33:373–380.

15. Rodriguez MA, Sheldon WR, Bauer HM, et al. The factors associated with disclosure of intimate partner abuse to clinicians. J Fam Pract 2001; 50(4):338–344.

16. Astbury J, Cabral M. Women's mental health: an evidence based review. Geneva: Mental Health Determinants and Populations, Department of Mental Health and Substance Dependence, World Health Organization; 2000, 121.

17. Rosenberg M, Fenley MA, Johnson D, et al. Bridging prevention and practice: public health and family violence. Acad Med 1997; 72(January Suppl. 1):S13–18.

18. Stark E, Flitcraft A. Women at risk: domestic violence and women's health. Thousand Oaks, CA: Sage; 1996.

19. Heise LL. Violence against women: an integrated, ecological framework. Violence Against Women 1998; 4(3):262–290.

20. Pinn VW, Chunko MT. The diverse faces of violence: minority women and domestic abuse. Acad Med 1997; 72(January Suppl. 1):S65–71.

21. Ellis MJ. Barriers to effective screening for domestic violence by Registered Nurses in the Emergency Department. Crit Care Nurs Q 1999; 22:27–41.

22. Walker L. Are personality disorders gender biased? In: Kirk SA, Einbinder SD, eds. Controversial issues in mental health. New York: Allyn and Bacon; 1994:21–29.

22. Richman J, Flaherry J. Gender differences in narcissistic styles. Psychiatry 1988; 51:368–377.

23. Dutton D, Browning J. Power struggles and intimacy anxieties as causative factors for violence in intimate relationships. In: Russell B, ed. Violence in intimate relationships. New York: Sage; 1987:163–175.

24. Fagan J, Browne A. Marital violence: physical aggression between women and men in intimate relationship. In: Reiss AJ Jr., Roth JA, eds. Understanding and preventing violence, Vol. 3: Social influences. Washington, DC: National Academy Press; 1994:115–292.

25. Candib L. Medicine and the family: a feminist perspective. New York: Harper Collins; 1995.

26. Kohut H. Introspection, empathy, and psychoanalysis: an examination of the relationship between mode of observation and theory. In: Ornstein P, ed. The search for the self. New York: International Universities Press; 1978:205–282.

27. Atwood G, Stolorow R. Structures of subjectivity: explorations in psychoanalytic phenomenology. Hillsdale, NJ: Analytic Press; 1984.

28. Guze PA. Cultivating curricular reform. Acad Med 1995; 70(11):971–973.

29. Ontario Medical Association curriculum guidelines for the medical management of wife abuse for undergraduate medical students. Toronto: Ontario Medical Association; 1990:9.

30. Hoff LA, Ross M. Violence content in nursing curricula: strategic issues and implementation. J Adv Nurs 1995; 21(1):137–142.

31. Alpert EJ. Interpersonal violence and the education of physicians. Acad Med 1997; 72(January Suppl. 1):S41–50.

32. Birrer RC, Vourkas C, Wang C, et al. Domestic violence: curricular issues in family medicine. In: Hamberger LK, Burge SK, Graham AV, et al., eds. Violence issues for health care educators and providers. Binghampton, NY: Haworth Trauma and Maltreatment Press; 1997:113–129.

33. Hamberger LK, Feuerbach SP, Borman RJ. Detecting the wife batterer. Med Aspects Hum Sex 1990; September:32–39.

34. Culross PL. Health care system responses to children exposed to domestic violence. Future Child 1999; 9(3):111–121.

35. Ferris LE, Norton P, Dunn EV, et al. Guidelines for managing domestic abuse when male and female partners are patients of the same physician. JAMA 1997; 278(10):851–857.

36. Felitti VJ, Anda RF, Nordenberg D, et al. Relationship of childhood abuse and household dysfunction to many of the leading causes of death in adults: the Adverse Childhood Experiences (ACE) Study. Am J Prev Med 1998; 14(4):245–258.

37. Dube SR, Anda RF, Felitti VJ, et al. Exposure to abuse, neglect, and household dysfunction among adults who witnessed intimate partner violence as children: implications for health and social services. Violence Vict 2002; 17(1):3–17.

38. McFarlane JM, Groff JY, O'Brien JA, et al. Behaviors of children who are exposed and not exposed to intimate partner violence: an analysis of 330 black, white, and Hispanic children. Pediatrics 2003; 112(3 Pt 1):202–207.

39. Wolfe DA, Crooks CV, Lee V, et al. The effects of children's exposure to domestic violence: a meta-analysis and critique. Clin Child Fam Psychol Rev 2003; 6(3):171–187.

40. Mintz H, Corbett F. When your patient is a batterer: what you need to know before treating perpetrators of domestic violence. Postgrad Med 1997; 101(3):219–21, 225–228.

41. Adams D. Guidelines for doctors on identifying and helping their patients who batter. J Am Med Womens Assoc 1996; 51(3):123–126.

42. Muelleman RL, Burgess P. Male victims of domestic violence and their history of perpetrating violence. Acad Emerg Med 1998; 5(9):866–870.

43. Berger RP, Bogen D, Dulani T, et al. Implementation of a program to teach pediatric residents and faculty about domestic violence. Arch Pediat Adol Med. 2002; 156(8):804–810.

44. Bair-Merritt MH, Giardino AP, Turner M, et al. Pediatric residency training on domestic violence: a national survey. Ambul Pediatr 2004; 4(1):24–27.

45. Holtrop TG, Fischer H, Gray SM, et al. Screening for domestic violence in a general pediatric clinic: be prepared! Pediatrics 2004; 114(5):1253.

46. Kassebaum DG. Proceedings of the AAMC's Consensus Conference on the Education of Medical Students about Family Violence and Abuse. Introduction: Why another conference on family violence?, and Conference Summary. Acad Med 1995; 70(11):961.

47. Short LM, Cotton D, Hodgson CS. Evaluation of the module on domestic violence at the UCLA School of Medicine. Acad Med 1997; 72(January Suppl. 1):S75–91.

48. Paluzzi P, Gaffikin L, Nanda J. The American College of Nurse-Midwives' Domestic Violence Education Project: evaluation and results. J Midwifery Womens Health 2000; 45(5):384–391.

49. Harris JM Jr., Kutob RM, Surprenant ZJ, et al. Can Internet-based education improve physician confidence in dealing with domestic violence? Fam Med 2002; 34(4):287–292.

50. Haist SA, Wilson JF, Pursley HG, et al. Domestic violence: increasing knowledge and improving skills with a four-hour workshop using standardized patients. Acad Med 2003; 78(10 Suppl. l):S24–26.

51. Thompson RS, Rivara FP, Thompson DC, et al. Identification and management of domestic violence: a randomized trial. Am J Prev Med 2000; 19(4):253–263.

52. Sugg NK, Inui T. Primary care physicians' response to domestic violence: opening Pandora's box. JAMA 1992; 267(23):3157–3160.

53. Warshaw C, Coffey V, Schultz B, et al. An advocacy based medical school elective on domestic violence. Poster presented at National Conference on Cultural Competence and Women's Health, Curricula in Medical Education. Washington, DC; 1995.

54. Ambuel B, Hamberger, LK, Lahti, J. The Family Peace Project: a model for training health care professionals to identify, treat and prevent partner violence. Waukesha, WI: Department of Family and Community Medicine, Medical College of Wisconsin; 1996.

55. Nicolaidis C. The voices of survivors documentary: using patient narrative to educate physicians about domestic violence. J Gen Intern Med 2002; 17(2):117–124.

56. Warshaw C, Riordan K. Domestic violence. In: Noble J, Greene HL, Levinson GA, et al., eds. Textbook of primary care medicine, 3rd edn. St. Louis: Mosby; 2001:497–504.

57. Mandel J, Marcotte D. Teaching family practice residents to identify and treat battered women. J Fam Pract 1983; 17(4):708–716.

58. Colliver JA, Swartz MH. Assessing clinical performance with standardised patients. JAMA 1997; 278(9):790–791.

59. Rieker P, Carmen E. The victim-to-patient process: the disconfirmation and transformation of abuse. Am J Orthopsychiatry 1986; 56:360–370.

60. Warshaw C, Ganley A, Salber P. Improving the health care response to domestic violence: a resource manual for health care providers. San Francisco: Family Violence Prevention Fund and Pennsylvania Coalition Against Domestic Violence; 1995.

61. Coeling HV, Harman G. Learning to ask about domestic violence. Womens Health Issues 1997; 7(4):263–267.

62. Bacchus L, Mezey G, Bewley S. Women's perceptions and experiences of routine enquiry for domestic violence in a maternity service. Brit J Obstet Gynaec 2002; 109:9–16.

63. Merritt-Gray M, Wuest J. Counteracting abuse and breaking free: the process of leaving revealed through women's voices. Health Care Women Int 1995; 16:399–412.

64. Bergman B, Brismar B, Nordin C. Utilisation of medical care by abused women. BMJ 1992; 305:27–29.

65. McCosker HM. Phenomenographic study of women's experiences of domestic violence during the childbearing years. Online Journal of Issues in Nursing; 2003. Available from: http://www.nursingworld.org/ojin/topic17/tpc_6.htm

66. Hayward KS, Weber LM. A community partnership to prepare nursing students to respond to domestic violence. Nurs Forum 2003; 38(3):5–10.

67. Mandel JB, Marcotte DB. Teaching family practice residents to identify and treat battered women. J Fam Pract 1983; 17(4):708–709, 715–716.

68. Power C. Converting the silence into action: the nurse's role in domestic violence. In: Gray G, Pratt R, eds. Issues in Australian Nursing 3. Melbourne: Churchill Livingstone; 1992:61–74.

69. Ernst A, Houry D, Weiss S, et al. Domestic violence awareness in a medical school class: 2-year follow-up. South Med J 2000; 93(8):772–776.

70. Zachary MJ, Schechter CB, Kaplan ML, et al. Provider evaluation of a multifaceted system of care to improve recognition and management of pregnant women experiencing domestic violence. Womens Health Issues 2002; 12(1):5–15.

71. Dutton MA. Empowering and healing the battered woman: a model for assessment and intervention. New York: Springer; 1992.

72. McCann IL, Pearlman LA. Vicarious retraumatization: a contextual model for understanding the effects of trauma on helper. J Trauma Stress 1990; 3:131–149.

73. deLahunta EA, Tulsky AA. Personal exposure of faculty and medical students to family violence. JAMA 1996; 275:1903–1906.

74. Miller T, Cohen M, Wiersman B. Crime in the United States: victim costs and consequences. Washington, DC: National Institute of Justice; 1995.

Chapter 5

Identification of intimate partner abuse in health care settings: should health professionals be screening?

Kelsey Hegarty, Gene Feder, and Jean Ramsay

On intake, I was asked all these screening questions and I was amazed and horrified to find myself answering 'yes', 'yes', 'yes', 'yes' to question after question. And it was then, at that moment, that I realized, 'My God, this does apply to me!'[1]

[Interviewer: Was it helpful to have people ask you?]

Oh yeah. It was real comforting to know that someone cared ... You knew the door was open.[2]

INTRODUCTION

Intimate partner abuse (IPA) is a hidden reality for many women attending health practitioners and in the wider community (see Chapter 2).[3-6] It is a substantial public health problem with major physical and psychological health consequences for women (see Chapter 3).[7] In contrast to the magnitude of the problem, there is consistent evidence that (a) the majority of women who are being abused by their partners do not disclose this to health professionals, and (b) that health professionals are reluctant to inquire about abuse.[3,8-11] As a result, only a minority of abused women are recognized in health care settings.[12] In a general practice-based study in the UK, only one in seven women with a history of domestic violence had any indication of abuse in their medical record.[3] However, we know from interviews with survivors of partner abuse that health professionals are the major professional group that women would want to tell and that this is a prerequisite for partner abuse interventions in health care settings.

This chapter will outline how women seek help and the barriers and facilitators to identification of IPA in health care settings, including the barriers to disclosure by women and inquiry by practitioners. The views of women and health professionals about inquiry, and women's views about what they want from health professionals, will be explored. We will examine recommendations for professionals about whom and how they should be asking about partner abuse. Finally, the current national and international debates around screening in health care settings will be discussed.

HEALTH SERVICES USED BY WOMEN EXPERIENCING IPA

There is a typical sequence of help-seeking behaviour followed by women experiencing partner abuse.[13] Women are unlikely to seek help after the first experience of abuse or violence from a partner. As the violence continues and escalates, although inhibiting factors of shame and embarrassment persist, women will attempt to seek help. Almost all women turn to families and friends first, although their abusive partner may have isolated them from potential sources of support. Only as the violence and abuse persists, especially in times of crisis, do they seek help from professional agencies: domestic violence organizations, police, lawyers, and health professionals. Small surveys have shown that general practitioners are often the first professional group to which women experiencing abuse turn to for help.[13,14] In an attempt to get help, women may also disclose to a range of other health and allied professionals: personal and relationship counsellors, child specialists, psychiatrists, psychologists, nurse practitioners, hospital staff, and family support workers. However, many women who experience partner abuse do not tell anyone about the abuse for months or years.

BARRIERS TO DISCLOSURE FROM THE WOMAN'S VIEWPOINT

The majority of women do not disclose abuse to health professionals, with lifetime disclosure rates varying from 18 to 37%.[9,15,16] In interview-[17-22] and survey-based studies,[5,9,11] women have reported many barriers to disclosure

Table 5.1   Barriers to disclosure by women of IPA

Internal barriers	External barriers
■ Embarrassment and shame ■ Denial or minimization of abuse ■ Emotional bonds to partner ■ Hope for change ■ Staying for the sake of the children ■ Normalization of violence ■ Fear of reprisal from their partners ■ Depression ■ Feeling that they will not be believed	■ Social isolation ■ Perception that services will not be able to help often due to previous unhelpful experiences ■ Perception that health professionals are there for physical problems only ■ Concern about confidentiality of information given to health professionals ■ Racism and culturally inappropriate services

at individual, family, and societal levels. Reasons given by women for not disclosing abuse can be understood from both an internal and an external perspective (see Table 5.1).[5,18,21,23,24]

Feeling ashamed, and/or a belief that it is their problem and that they should be able to manage it themselves, are barriers to disclosure for many abused women. This reflects wider community beliefs about the 'privacy' of the family,[25] reinforced by responses from health practitioners that deny or minimize the abuse or imply that the woman is responsible for provoking it.[22,24] Other women may not wish to confide in health professionals who are also providing care for their partner. Some women, while not assuming that a health professional will be hostile to disclosure, assume that partner abuse falls outside their professional remit, which is perceived to be largely medical and health problems. Finally, women experiencing abuse may judge that disclosure to health professionals will not improve their situation and may even expose them to greater risk from potential breaches in confidentiality.[21]

Culturally inappropriate support services are another obvious barrier for women from a non-English-speaking background (see Chapter 11). Indigenous women (see Chapter 12) describe racism as the main structural barrier to disclosure. Thus there are many internal and external barriers that stop women disclosing IPA to health professionals.

BARRIERS TO INQUIRY FROM THE HEALTH PROFESSIONAL'S VIEWPOINT

Health professionals frequently fail to inquire about IPA, with rates of inquiry varying from 13 to 20%.[8–10,15,26–29] Furthermore, physicians and nurses often fail to document physical violence in medical records.[3] Waalen and colleagues[30] reviewed 12 quantitative studies that identified barriers to IPA screening as perceived by health care providers. The main provider-related barriers include:

■ lack of provider education regarding partner abuse;
■ lack of time;
■ lack of effective interventions.

Respondents in the primary studies frequently cited patient-related factors, such as non-disclosure and fear of offending the patient.[31] The review[30] concluded that barriers to screening for IPA are similar among health care providers across diverse specialties and settings.

These barriers arise from failures in undergraduate and postgraduate training, and from structural problems within health care systems, as well as from attitudes of individual health professionals. Coverage of domestic violence is either absent or marginal in the training of health professionals, which reflects an implicit view that IPA in particular, and gender inequality in general, are not health issues.[19,32]

One of the main structural barriers is limited time within consultations and health care settings. Partner abuse often requires the health professional to deal with a number of outside agencies and organizations, which can be both time consuming and frustrating.[33]

Health practitioners frequently hold attitudes that prevent them from addressing the problem. Complementing quantitative surveys, several interview studies[19,34,35] have also explored the barriers to identification of IPA. Health professionals hesitate to inquire about abusive experiences in their patients' lives because they feel helpless to intervene. In the absence of training, the professional may advise a woman disclosing abuse to leave her abusive partner. As she may be unable to, or choose not to do so, the professional feels there is little else to offer and becomes frustrated. A frequently quoted phrase is that they are reluctant to 'open Pandoras Box'.[35] Health professionals often fear offending the patient by inquiring into such a 'private matter'.[19,27,35] For some, the acknowledgement of violence may raise the issue of abuse in their own family.[33,34]

Brown and colleagues[19] reported that gender issues were identified by some health practitioners as being a barrier, in that some of the male doctors felt incapable of dealing with this issue. One interview study in the US[36] attempted to explore the difference between doctors' and nurses' responses to domestic violence. They found that women professionals, regardless of profession, were more sympathetic than men towards abused women. An additional barrier for general practitioners is that the perpetrator may also be their patient.[37] This creates a conflict for the doctor, who feels they cannot 'take sides', reflecting a widely held societal belief about violence against a partner being a private matter and not unacceptable criminal behaviour.

FACILITATION OF DISCLOSURE TO HEALTH PROFESSIONALS

Gerbert[38] interviewed women who had experienced abuse from their partners and describes 'the complicated dance of disclosure by victims and identification by health care providers'. The decision to disclose abuse to a health professional is complex and women will choose when and to whom to disclose, if to anyone. This decision will be influenced by the nature of the abuse, the woman's perception of her needs, her trust (or lack of trust) in the health professional's ability to respond appropriately, and the way that the health professional asks about abuse.

Factors that positively influence women to disclose partner abuse include a perception of the health professional as sympathetic, able to listen to her problems, able to maintain confidentiality, and having the potential to help.[24] Good communication skills of the health professional facilitate disclosure.[39] However, whilst the explicit inquiry by the health professional is associated with a greater disclosure rate, women are rarely asked in clinical consultations.[9]

Women who reported disclosing abuse in a general practice-based study, when compared with women who had not disclosed, were almost twice as likely to be middle aged, to have experienced combined (physical, emotional, and sexual) abuse during their lifetime, or to be afraid of their partner.[9] Women who self-rated as experiencing a 'little' or 'some' abuse were significantly less likely to disclose than women who perceived they had experienced 'moderate' or 'great' abuse. Overall, women's own perception of the abuse, the severity of the abuse, and the communication skills of the health professional appear to be the key factors in facilitation of disclosure.

HOW SHOULD HEALTH PROFESSIONALS IDENTIFY WOMEN WHO EXPERIENCE IPA?

Earlier recommendations by organizations such as the American Medical Association (1992) to screen all women presenting to primary care has caused heated debate amongst researchers and practitioners.[40,41] Gerbert[38] points out that although screening questions and guidelines have been developed for health professionals, these guidelines often fail to address the complexity of the interaction between women and their health care providers. Furthermore, the guidelines give little insight into how health professionals can overcome the patient and professional barriers to identification. In a focus group study of obstetricians, gynaecologists, and emergency department and primary care physicians ($n = 45$) who had expertise in approaching the identification of victims, five themes emerged:

- how experienced professionals framed questions to reduce patient discomfort;
- patient cues that prompted them to suspect IPA;
- direct and indirect approaches to identification with an emphasis on facilitating patient trust and disclosure over time;
- direct patient disclosure is rare;
- how experienced professionals redefined successful outcomes of universal screening.

Each of these will be dealt with in the sections below, before we turn to the issue of universal screening.

How should health professionals ask about abuse?

Questions need to be carefully framed and sensitively asked to minimize patient discomfort. Sensitive inquiry is likely to elicit disclosure[24] and the challenge for health professionals is to pose questions about safety and fear of partners in an appropriate way with women who are experiencing partner abuse in their lives.

Over the last 10 years, researchers have developed and evaluated different sets of questions about partner abuse to ask in clinical settings.[42–45] There is insufficient evidence to recommend for or against the use of a specific set of questions or screening instrument.[46] Furthermore, we concur with Lachs'[47] wry comment: 'investigators seeking the colonoscopic equivalent of a domestic abuse screening test may well be on a fool's errand'. It is very unlikely that a single question will cover the range of women's experiences of partner abuse; e.g. women with disabilities, indigenous women, women in lesbian relationships, and women of non-English-speaking backgrounds. Moreover, the temperament of the professional and their personal consulting style will make some formulations more appropriate then others. Box 5.1 gives examples of how professionals can frame initial questions about partner abuse.

Box 5.1   Possible questions to ask and statements to make if you suspect IPA

- Has your partner ever physically threatened or hurt you?
- Is there a lot of tension in your relationship?
- Sometimes partners react strongly in arguments and use physical force. Is this happening to you?
- Are you afraid of your partner?
- Have you ever been afraid of any partner?
- Violence is very common in the home. I ask a lot of my patients about abuse because no one should have to live in fear of their partners.

What patient cues should alert health professionals to suspect abuse?

When women present with the symptoms or clinical conditions associated with abuse, such as injuries, pelvic pain, vaginal discharge, depression, anxiety, or irritable bowel syndrome (see Chapter 3),[5,7,48] or with a history of IPA in their family, health practitioners should think of partner abuse. However, many practitioners forget that IPA can be an underlying cause[38] of unexplained symptoms or clinical conditions (overall these are poor predictors of IPA[49,50]). Health practitioners should also watch for signs in women's body language and listen for hints and discrepancies that signal partial disclosure.[38]

Validation role of inquiry through direct and indirect approaches

Inquiry by a health professional about partner abuse may signal to a woman that it is unacceptable and that her feelings about it are valid. This possibility has not been adequately investigated. However, in interview studies, women describe that being asked about abuse, even if they choose not to disclose, gives the message that IPA is unacceptable and that their feelings are valid. This validation extends to the response of health professionals once a woman has disclosed.[38] Health professionals experienced in dealing with partner abuse say that development of a trusting relationship with patients over time and indirect non-judgemental validation are central to facilitation of disclosure by patients.[18,38] As we explore further in Chapter 6, health care settings, particularly those where there is a potential long-term relationship between women and health professionals, may be the only places where a woman feels safe to discuss partner abuse and have her feelings validated. Clear validating messages that health practitioners could use are shown in Box 5.2.

Box 5.2 Possible validation statements if a woman discloses IPA[53]

- Everybody deserves to feel safe at home.
- You don't deserve to be hit or hurt and it is not your fault.
- This is not your fault, you didn't cause this.
- I am concerned about your safety and well-being.
- You are not alone, I will be with you through this, whatever you decide. Help is available.
- You are my patient; I know you are suffering. I care about you. You may not have seen me as someone to help you solve this problem, but I am ready to help you to the best of my ability now or in the future.[47]
- You are not to blame. Abuse is common and happens in all kinds of relationships. It tends to continue.
- Abuse can affect your health and that of your children in many ways.

Direct patient disclosure is rare

This chapter has highlighted the low levels of patient disclosure to practitioners. Health practitioners need to respect women's situations and choices about disclosure, whilst still offering ongoing support for a woman in the hope that she feels it is safe and appropriate to disclose at a future visit.

Health care providers redefine successful outcomes of universal screening

Some health practitioners have come to believe that successful screening for, or inquiry about, IPA needs to be redefined so that compassionate asking is an end in itself, independent of disclosure.[38] In any discussion on when to ask about abuse, it is important to distinguish between *universal screening* (the application of a standardized question to all symptom-free women according to a procedure that does not vary from place to place) and *case finding* (asking questions if indicators are present).[39] We have already argued that clinical indicators may be poor predictors of abuse. Therefore, Taket and colleagues[51] argue that a strong case exists for *routinely inquiring* about partner abuse in many health care settings because the rates of disclosure without direct questioning in health care settings are poor.[52] Among the authors of that paper there was a range of views about the meaning of 'routine inquiry'. At one end of the spectrum, there was a view that it essentially meant asking all women within health care settings; in effect, a screening programme. At the other end, there was a view that it meant having a low threshold for asking women in clinical consultations, nearer to case finding. The clinicians in the group tended towards the case finding end of the spectrum. If health practitioners routinely ask about IPA, this can be seen as a validating message that it is a health care issue, regardless of patient disclosure.[53]

What do women and health professionals think about screening?

A recent systematic review examined the acceptability of screening by health professionals, both from the perspective of women attending health care services and from the viewpoint of the clinicians themselves.[54] In the four American studies reviewed that elicited the views of women patients about screening, the response was generally positive. In two of the studies three-quarters or more of the women thought that routine screening was acceptable, whereas in the remaining two studies just under half of all women found it acceptable. Furthermore, the views of respondents who were abused or not abused were largely similar, although in one of the primary studies abused women were significantly more in favour of screening than non-abused women.[55] Health professionals were more ambivalent about screening in the two primary studies in the review. In the first, where the views of primary care physicians in New England were sought[56], 33% responded that they were in favour of routine screening. The second study, also conducted in the US, elicited the attitudes of accident and emergency department nurses. Fifty-three per cent of respondents said they thought that nurses should routinely screen all women for a history of domestic violence.[54]

A recent survey of maternity units in Scotland found that only 15% of midwives routinely inquired about domestic violence whilst only 45% did so even when there were indications.[57] Similarly, a British study found 55% of midwives disagreed with questions about domestic violence being part of routine care.[58] Horan and colleagues[28] surveyed 662 obstetricians and found that 37% screened during pregnancy for domestic violence. An in-depth focus group study of midwives suggests that, even if they are enthusiastic about implementing screening, there are a range of difficulties when it comes to putting screening into practice.[34] Lack of time means that midwives found it difficult to implement the screening and they often felt poorly equipped to deal with this social problem.

On the basis of these and other findings, it appears that screening by health professionals does increase the identification of domestic violence and that many women do not object to being asked routinely.[54] However, the majority of health professionals appear not to be in favour of screening of women in health care settings.

SHOULD HEALTH CARE PROFESSIONALS BE SCREENING?

If we attempt to apply the medical and public health model of screening to IPA, there are some problematic issues (see Box 5.3). Although IPA is common and causes major morbidity and mortality, we are relatively ignorant about the natural history of partner abuse. Survivors of violence and abuse do not have asymptomatic disease they are hoping to have detected in a pre-clinical state, like early cancer patients.[47] Furthermore, as discussed in the inquiry section above, the issues involved in finding a screening test that has minimal misidentification when there is no universal definition (see Chapter 2) of what constitutes IPA are great.

Box 5.3   World Health Organization screening criteria

- An important health problem.
- Natural history is well understood.
- Identifiable early stage for intervention.
- Suitable screening test available.
- Test acceptable to women.
- Satisfactory diagnostic test with agreed case definition.
- Effective management for the recognized condition.
- Resources required acceptable and feasible to benefits.

Finally, before advising health professionals to screen every woman for partner abuse, it must first be established that screening does more good than harm. The Canadian Task Force on Preventive Health Care has concluded that there is insufficient evidence to recommend for or against routine screening for violence against women.[59] The US Preventive Service Task Force found essentially no studies of reasonable quality supporting effective interventions for intimate partner violence.[60] We have no evidence that women will have better outcomes from any interventions in primary care.[54,61]

However, as Lachs[47] points out, it is hard to acknowledge how prevalent IPA is in clinical practice and simply conclude that we should do nothing because there is currently no proof. Bradley and colleagues[8] suggest that questioning 'should be thought of as a way of uncovering and reframing a hidden stigma'. Asking in whatever way makes the health professional and woman feel comfortable, and responding in a non-judgemental way may be all we can offer. Although there are only a small number of studies that have measured health outcomes for women resulting from interventions in the health care setting (see Chapter 6), interview studies suggest that there is a benefit for women in accessing specialized support services.[51]

Other professionals, however, challenge the assumption that disclosure of intimate partner violence is always beneficial to women[62] and have concerns about individuals trying to implement screening interventions in health care settings without sufficient training, support, and resources, resulting in well-motivated changes that may have harmful outcomes. García-Moreno[39] calls for clearer guidelines on 'who should ask the questions, of whom, in which settings, and after what training'. The National Consensus Guidelines from the Family Violence Prevention Fund in the US emphasizes the issues of prerequisite training for health professionals. Before *screening or routine inquiry* is instituted in a health care setting, health professionals require training (see Chapter 4) to enable them to sensitively inquire and provide appropriate advice and options for women who disclose abuse and violence.[37] Assessing and ensuring the safety of women and children during and after disclosure is a high priority in any debate on screening in health care settings (see Box 5.4).

Box 5.4   Assessment of immediate safety

- Are you in immediate danger?
- Do you want to go home today to your partner?
- Do you have somewhere safe to go?
- Has the violence got worse or is it getting scarier?
- Has your partner used weapons?
- Has your partner ever held you/your children against your will?
- Does your partner ever watch you closely or follow you?
- Has your partner ever threatened to kill you, themselves or your children?

(Adapted from National Consensus Guidelines, Family Violence Prevention Fund, US)

CONCLUSION

Women who have experienced IPA describe waiting to be asked by caring health providers who communicate well in a confidential manner.[24,51,63] Health professionals need to be aware of the likelihood of abuse in women's lives and have the skills to ask sensitively about abuse and fear of their partners and be able to appropriately support and advocate for them. Candib[64] urges us to go even further and think about asking men about their use of violence in their relationships and to work with parents and children regarding issues of control and violence. It is documented that the cost of domestic violence to the community[65] is high in health utilization and in women's and children's lives. Health professionals should have a low threshold for sensitively asking the hard questions about fear, control, and abuse with women and with men that they see in clinical practice.

Health professional education programmes should emphasize relevant communication skills and attitudes, particularly in sensitive psychosocial areas, at undergraduate, postgraduate, and continuing education levels to ensure women have access to appropriate care. Health professionals need education and support to be sufficiently confident to ask women patients about current or past abuse. There is insufficient evidence of effectiveness or even the absence of harm to implement screening programmes for partner abuse in health care settings, but professionals need to be alert to cues (both overt and hidden) that women consulting them may be experiencing violence and abuse. Women who are young, have recently separated or divorced, are pregnant, or are presenting with psychological symptoms are particularly vulnerable. There is already some evidence that specific interventions, such as advocacy may benefit women who have recently experienced abuse, but we believe that policy in this area needs to be informed by more robust research, including well-designed randomized trials (see

Chapter 6). Health professionals must be supported with knowledge based on good evidence and appropriate skills to manage the consequences of abuse and violence in women's lives if we are going to help improve health outcomes for women and their children.

REFERENCES

1. Nicolaidis CT. The voices of survivors documentary: using patient narrative to educate physicians about domestic violence. J Gen Intern Med 2002; 17:117–124.
2. Zink T, Elder N, Jacobson J, et al. Medical management of intimate partner violence considering the stages of change: precontemplation and contemplation. Ann Fam Med 2004; 2:231–239.
3. Richardson J, Coid J, Petruckevitch A, et al. Identifying domestic violence: cross sectional study in primary care. BMJ 2002; 324:1–6.
4. Watts C, Zimmerman C. Violence against women: global scope and magnitude. Lancet 2002; 359:1232–1237.
5. McCauley J, Kern DE, Kolodner K, et al. The 'battering syndrome': prevalence and clinical characteristics of domestic violence in primary care internal medicine practices. Ann Intern Med 1995; 123:737–746.
6. McLennan W. Women's Safety Survey. Canberra: Australian Bureau of Statistics; 1996.
7. Campbell JC. Health consequences of intimate partner violence. Lancet 2002; 359:1331–1336.
8. Bradley F, Smith M, Long J, et al. Reported frequency of domestic violence: cross sectional survey of women attending general practice. BMJ 2002; 324:1–6.
9. Hegarty K, Bush R. Prevalence of partner abuse in women attending Australian General Practice: a cross-sectional survey. Aust N Z J Public Health 2002; 26(5):437–442.
10. Hamberger LK, Saunders DG, Hovey M. Prevalence of domestic violence in community practice and rate of physician inquiry. Fam Med 1992; 24:283–287.
11. Mazza DL, Dennerstein L, Ryan V. Physical, sexual and emotional violence against women: a general practice-based prevalence study. Med J Aust 1996; 164:14–17.
12. Stark E, Flitcraft A. Women at risk: domestic violence and women's health. London: Sage; 1996.
13. Smith M. The incidence and prevalence of woman abuse in Toronto. Violence Vict 1987; 2:173–187.
14. Mazza D, Lawrence JM, Roberts GL, et al. What can we do about domestic violence? Med J Aust 2000; 173(10):532–535.
15. McGrath M, Hogan J, Peipert JF. A prevalence survey of abuse and screening for abuse in urgent care patients. Obstet Gynecol 1998; 91(4):511–514.
16. Swahnberg K, Wijma B, Schei B, et al. Are sociodemographic and regional and sample factors associated with prevalence of abuse? Acta Obstet Gynecol Scand 2004; 83:276–288.
17. Gerbert B, Johnston K, Caspers N, et al. Experiences of battered women in health care settings: a qualitative study. Women Health 1996; 24(3):1–14.
18. Head C, Taft A. Improving general practitioner management of women experiencing domestic violence: a study of the beliefs and experiences of women victim/survivors and of GPs. Canberra: Department of Health, Housing and Community Service; 1995.
19. Brown J, Lent B, Sas G. Identifying and treating wife abuse. J Fam Practice 1993; 36(2):185–191.
20. McMurray A, Moore K. Domestic violence: are we listening? Do we see? Aust J Adv Nurs 1994; 12(1):23–28.
21. Rodriguez M, Sheldon W, Bauer H, et al. The factors associated with disclosure of intimate partner abuse to clinicians. J Fam Practice 2001; 50(4):338–344.
22. Lutenbacher M, Coohlen A, Mitzel J. Do we really help? Perspectives of abused women. Public Health Nurs 2003; 20(1):56–64.
23. Keys Young. Against the odds: how women survive domestic violence. Canberra: Office of Status of Women; 1998.

24. Hegarty K, Taft A. Overcoming the barriers to disclosure and inquiry of partner abuse for women attending general practice. Aust N Z J Public Health 2001; 25(5):433–438.
25. ANOP Research Services. Community attitudes of violence against women. Canberra: Office of Status of Women; 1995.
26. Abbott J, Johnson R, Koziol-Mclain J, et al. Domestic violence against women: incidence and prevalence in an emergency department population. JAMA 1995; 273(22):1763–1767.
27. Parsons LH, Zaccaro D, Wells B, et al. Methods of and attitudes toward screening obstetrics and gynecology patients for domestic violence. Am J Obstet Gynecol 1995; 173:381–387.
28. Horan DL, Chapin J, Klein L, et al. Domestic violence screening practices of obstetri-cian-gynecologists. Obstet Gynecol 1998; 92(5):785–789.
29. Ellis MJ. Barriers to effective screening for domestic violence by registered nurses in the emergency department. Crit Care Nurs Q 1999; 22:27–41.
30. Waalen J, Goodwin M, Spitz A, et al. Screening for intimate partner violence by health care providers: barriers and interventions. Am J Prev Med 2000; 19(4):230–237.
31. Rodriguez MA, Bauer HM, McLoughlin E, et al. Screening and intervention for inti-mate partner abuse: practices and attitudes of primary care physicians. JAMA 1999; 282(5):468–474.
32. Warshaw C. Limitations of the medical model in the care of battered women. Gend Soc 1989; 3(4):506–517.
33. Candib LM. Violence against women: no more excuses. Fam Med 1989; 21(5):339–341.
34. Mezey G, Bacchus L, Haworth A, et al. Midwives' perceptions and experiences of routine enquiry for domestic violence. Brit J Obstet Gynaec 2003; 110:744–752.
35. Sugg NK, Inui T. Primary care physicians response to domestic violence. JAMA 1992; 267(23):3157–3160.
36. Rose K, Saunders DG. Nurses and physicians attitudes about women abuse: the effects of gender and professional role. Health Care Women Int 1986; 7:427–438.
37. Taft A, Broom D, Legge D. General practitioner management of intimate partner abuse and the whole family: a qualitative study. BMJ 2004; 328:618–621.
38. Gerbert B. How health care providers help battered women: the survivor's perspec-tive. Women Health 1999; 29:115–135.
39. Garcia-Moreno C, Watts C, Jansen H, et al. Responding to violence against women: a WHO multi-country study. Lancet 2002; 359:1232–1237.
40. Jewkes R. Intimate partner violence: causes and prevention. Lancet 2002; 359:1423–1429.
41. Cole T. Is domestic violence screening helpful? JAMA 2000; 284:551–553.
42. McFarlane J, Parker B, Soeken K, et al. Assessing for abuse during pregnancy: sever-ity and frequency of injuries and associated entry into prenatal care. JAMA 1992; 267(23):3176–3178.
43. Brown JLB, Schmidt G, Sas G. Application of the Woman Abuse Screening Tool (WAST) and WAST-Short in the family practice setting. J Fam Practice 2000; 49:896–903.
44. Sherin KM, Sinacore J, Li X, et al. HITS: a short domestic violence screening tool for use in a family practice setting. Fam Med 1998; 30(7):508–512.
45. Coker AL. Frequency and correlates of intimate partner violence by type: physical, sexual and psychological battering. Am J Public Health 2000; 90(4):553–559.
46. Thompson RS, Rivaro FP, Thompson DC, et al. Identification and management of domestic violence: a randomized trial. Am J Prev Med 2000; 19:253–263.
47. Lachs MS. Screening for family violence: what's an evidence-based doctor to do? Ann Intern Med 2004; 140(5):399–400.
48. Eisenstat S, Bancroft L. Domestic violence. New Engl J Med 1999; 341(12):886–892.
49. Zachary M, Mulvihill M, Burton W, et al. Domestic abuse in the emergency depart-ment: can a risk profile be defined? Acad Emerg Med 2001; 8:796–803.
50. Fanslow J, Norton R, Spinola C. Indicators of assault-related injuries among women presenting to the emergency department. Ann Emerg Med 1998; 32:341–348.
51. Taket A, Nurse J, Smith K, et al. Routinely asking women about domestic violence in health settings. BMJ 2003; 327(7416):673–676.
52. McLeer SV, Anwar R, Herman S, et al. Education is not enough: a systems failure in protecting battered women. Ann Emerg Med 1989; 18(6):651–653.

53. Gerbert B, Moe J, Caspers N, et al. Physicians' response to victims of domestic violence: toward a model of care. Women Health 2002; 35(2/3):1–22.

54. Gielen AC, O'Campo PJ, Campbell JC, et al. Women's opinions about domestic violence screening and mandatory reporting. Am J Prev Med 2000; 19:279–285.

55. Friedman L, Samet J, Roberts M, et al. Inquiry about victimisation experiences: a survey of patient preferences and physician practices. Arch Intern Med 1992; 152(June):1186–1190.

56. Foy R, Nelson F, Penney G, et al. Antenatal detection of domestic violence. Lancet 2000; 355:9218.

57. Scobie J, McGuire M. The silent enemy: domestic violence in pregnancy. Brit J Midwifery 1999; 7(4):259–262.

58. Ramsay J, Richardson J, Carter Y, et al. Should health professionals screen women for domestic violence? Systematic review. BMJ 2002; 325(7359):314.

59. MacMillan HL, Wathen CN, with the Canadian Task Force on Preventive Health Care. Prevention and treatment of violence against women: systematic review and recommendations. London, ON; Canadian Task Force on Preventive Health Care (CTFPHC) Technical Report 01–4. September 2001.

60. Nelson HD, Nguyen P, McInerney Y, et al. Screening women and elderly adults for family and intimate partner violence: a review of the evidence for the US Preventive Services Task Force. Ann Intern Med 2004; 140:382–386.

61. Wathen CN, MacMillan HL. Scientific review and clinical applications. Interventions for violence against women: scientific review. JAMA 2003; 289(5):589–600.

62. Hegarty K, Gunn J, Chondros P, et al. Association between depression and abuse by partners of women attending general practice: descriptive, cross sectional survey. BMJ 2004; 328(7440):621–624.

63 Fogarty C, Burge S, McCord EC. Communicating with patients about intimate partner violence: screening and interviewing approaches. Fam Med 2002; 34(5):369–375.

64. Candib L. Primary violence prevention. J Fam Practice 2000; 49:904–906.

65. Roberts G. Domestic violence: costing of service provision for female victims – 20 case histories. Brisbane: Department of Family Services; 1988.

Chapter 6

Clinician response to women experiencing intimate partner abuse: what is the evidence for good practice and policy?

Gene Feder, Jean Ramsay, and Mary Zachary

She didn't make it seem like she was shocked. She was very understanding and she didn't ask me questions like 'why did you let him do this'. She didn't judge me.[1]

Just compassion is going to open one door. And when we feel safe and are able to trust, that makes a hell of a lot of difference as compared with being run through the system.[1]

INTRODUCTION

This chapter reviews research that should inform the development of good practice by clinicians towards women with a recent experience of partner abuse.

We review evidence about support to women by clinicians and about interventions based on advocacy, protocols, and training. We also explore the importance of compassion and support by clinicians to whom women disclose abuse and the importance of embedding good practice in health care settings into a wider community response to partner abuse. We conclude by highlighting key recommendations in a selection of current national health care guidelines on domestic violence. The problematic nature of the evidence underpinning health care policy on partner abuse is explored in the final chapter.

SOURCES OF EVIDENCE AND SCOPE OF THIS CHAPTER

This chapter is largely based on the studies identified in five systematic reviews[2-6] that have restricted their inclusion criteria to quantitative studies (see Table 6.1). We have included studies that evaluate interventions for women who are experiencing current abuse. Clinicians also have a role in responding to women with past abuse, but that is not the focus of this chapter.

In our overview of the evidence we are particularly interested in studies of interventions in health care settings, as these are most directly relevant to clinicians. We have also included studies of interventions in other settings to which clinicians can refer women who disclose abuse to them. We are not reporting on the totality of studies included in the reviews, and refer the reader to the cited papers or book chapters if they want to understand the scope and methodological limitations of the primary studies and to pursue the evidence base in more detail. For information about the content and setting of specific interventions it is necessary to consult the papers reporting the primary studies.

The interventions aim largely at secondary prevention: preventing further abuse. Primary prevention – preventing the onset of abuse – is a larger political and cultural challenge to which health services do not directly contribute, other than reflecting the unacceptability of partner abuse. Tertiary prevention – dealing with the consequences of abuse once abuse has ceased – overlaps with secondary prevention and we address this to some extent in our section on psychological interventions. The distinction between secondary and tertiary prevention is not clear-cut, as abuse often recurs and intensifies after a woman leaves an abusive relationship.

What about screening?

A controversial question about good practice in health care settings is whether the implementation of screening programmes is justified. This issue is tackled in a separate chapter (Chapter 5). To some extent questions about effectiveness of interventions to improve outcomes for women experiencing

Table 6.1   Systematic reviews of partner abuse interventions relevant to health care

Review first author and date	Searched for primary studies or reviews until	Inclusion criteria	Number of studies
Davidson[5]	2000	English language; published and unpublished studies on treatment interventions in health care settings for domestic violence	3
Ramsay[4]	February 2001	English and French; published controlled on interventions in health care settings	6
Wathen[2]	March 2002	? language restrictions; comparative studies evaluating interventions to which a primary care clinician could refer a patient, including interventions for perpetrators	22
Klevens[3]	November 2002	No language restriction. Controlled studies of interventions initiated in health care settings	11
Abel[6]	1996	Any study measuring outcomes of psychosocial treatments	9

abuse have been overshadowed by the debate over screening.[4,7] Although settling this debate requires consideration of the effectiveness of interventions that result from screening, judgements about interventions are independent of how women are identified. This separation between screening and interventions is complicated by the fact that screening or routine questioning of women in health care settings is an intervention in its own right. The act of asking a woman about abuse, signalling that abuse is a health care issue that can be talked about, and thereby legitimating and eliciting disclosure, can have a powerful effect on a woman who has not been able to tell anyone about her situation.[7]

A CONCEPTUAL MODEL

Most of the interventions that we describe below are not explicitly based on a conceptual framework or model. Such models are useful for contextualizing interventions and to inform research and implementation. Theory-based approaches to interventions for domestic violence exist, but remain largely untested.[8] A greater body of work exists on conceptual frameworks for understanding the causes, dynamics, and effects of abuse, as discussed in Chapters 1, 2, and 3. These can help us formulate conceptual frameworks for interventions.

We think it is particularly important to articulate a broader conceptual model within which to locate specific interventions, because of the danger of isolating health care-based interventions from essential community, family, and individual efforts for realizing the safety of women experiencing abuse. This is true for other complex public health problems, like childhood accidents or prevention of tuberculosis, but is amplified in the case of partner abuse by the lack of control women have over their abusive partner's actions and lack of resources to ensure their safety and that of their children. Furthermore, a woman is at increased risk of abuse when she attempts to separate from her partner; this reinforces the need for planned collaboration between health, legal, police, and social services involvement.

We believe that intervention at three levels is needed in partner violence programmes that are based in, or include, health care organizations:

- community/environmental/political level;
- health care organization level;
- individual/family/social support level.

All are important for creating a community-wide response that effectively addresses the needs of survivors and stops further abuse by the perpetrator. Conceptual frameworks are needed that operate in each dimension. We are not aware of any models that adequately address each dimension.

Theoretical constructs that underpin the individual, health care setting, and community dimensions of domestic violence interventions exist. Among these are empowerment theory[9] for the individual/family/social support level, systems theory for organizational change, and a framework of community-coordinated response. The coordinated community response is an overarching concept based on an *a priori* assumption that community-based efforts must work as a coordinated system to assure the safety and well-being of women and their children. The model depicted in Fig. 6.1, originally articulated by Mary Zachary, connects individuals and health care systems to a community-wide response to partner violence. Within that framework of community participation, system-based interventions in health care settings are a widely accepted basis for implementing change in these settings, and empowerment theory is an individual approach to advocacy and counselling.

These dimensions provide a framework for our discussion on current evidence for the effectiveness of domestic violence interventions. The sides of the figure represent the underlying principles of confidentiality and

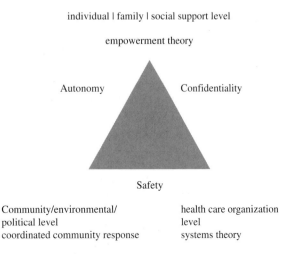

Figure 6.1 Empowerment theory.

autonomous decision making, while affirming safety as the overall goal of interventions.

VALIDATION OF WOMEN'S EXPERIENCES AND SUPPORT

The immediate response of clinicians to disclosure of abuse has not previously been characterized as an intervention and has not been the subject of controlled studies. We believe that it is a crucial part of what we have to offer women experiencing domestic violence. Health care settings, particularly those where there is a potential long-term relationship between women and health professionals (family practice, gynaecology, internal medicine, nurse practitioner practice), may be the only places where a woman feels safe to discuss partner abuse. If the experience of partner abuse is akin to being trapped in a war zone, disclosure to a doctor or nurse who knows you and responds compassionately can be, at least, a momentary escape and, at best, a step towards freedom. We know from interviews with survivors of partner abuse in California that women hope that their physicians and, presumably, other clinicians will respond to disclosure with unconditional support and no pressure to act in a particular way.[10] Physicians with expertise in domestic violence validate the experience of abuse that a woman discloses to them, affirm the unacceptability of that experience, and express solidarity, before any other response.[11] There are several key messages that we should try to convey when a woman has disclosed partner abuse:

- you believe her and are glad she told you;
- domestic violence is a crime: she has the right to report it;
- she is not alone: one in four women experience it at some point in their lives;
- she does not deserve it; her safety in her own home is a priority;
- her children are at risk;
- the abuser is responsible; his violence is not her fault;
- she has the right to feel the way she does, and talk about it;
- there is help available from other agencies and you can refer her.

Even if a woman does not choose to engage with outside agencies, validation of her experience by the health care professional and the offer of support is a moral and political act that may in the long run contribute to the woman being able to change her situation.

Much has been written on the experience of survivors and their expectations of health care workers, mostly emphasizing the process of screening and disclosure. In addition to offering support, the health care professional needs to make an assessment of the abused woman's safety. This may be as simple as checking with the woman that it is safe for her and her children, if she has any, to return home. A more detailed risk assessment will include questions about escalation of abuse, the content of threats, and direct and indirect abuse to the children.

The guidelines we discuss at the end of this chapter highlight the importance of the initial response of clinicians to women who disclose abuse, and give more details. Within the terms of the model presented in Fig. 6.1, validation and the expression of support is located at the individual level, promoting empowerment of the women disclosing abuse.

Ambiguous terminology makes comparison between studies difficult

The primary studies that constitute the evidence base for this chapter come from a range of disciplines (including clinical psychology, social work, nursing, and medicine) and countries, mostly from the United States, Australia, and New Zealand. Inevitably this means that the same terms are used differently in these studies. In particular, there is marked heterogeneity in the meaning of 'advocacy'. In most of the papers the authors do not define the term or describe their activity in any detail. An important distinction is between interventions that have a formal psychological component and those that provide support and information about community services. As would be expected in a field where community-based organizations and political advocates created the original response and continue to lead service efforts, terminology taken up by medical systems and psychiatric providers can be confusing. Advocates generally refer to individuals providing support and access to resources in the community, while advocacy as an activity should not be confined to specialist providers. Depending on the health care institution, in the United States counselling may refer to empathetic support in the context of education and referrals, or formal psychological treatment. In Australia and the United Kingdom, counselling entails psychological treatment, using a range of models. This ambiguity is compounded by the variety of roles and backgrounds of those engaged in advocacy and counselling. In the United States, social workers in community-based organizations may be referred to as advocates, while in other settings they may provide counselling based on psychiatric treatment paradigms. Conversely, advocates may have little formal training, but extensive experience in the field, and can work in either community or health care settings. The role of domestic violence advocates in health care settings overlaps with care coordinators or others with responsibility for coordinating domestic violence services. Another permutation of the advocate role is the training of lay women to give support to young mothers (see Chapter 7).

ADVOCACY

Domestic violence advocates, sometimes based in health care settings, but often in voluntary organizations in the community, accept self-referrals or clinician referrals. As we have discussed above, their roles vary between and within countries. Yet we can characterize their core role as providing information on legal, housing, and financial options and, crucially in the intervention studies we review here, *facilitating access and use of community resources* such as refuges or shelters, emergency housing, and psychological interventions. Depending on the specific advocacy model, and this is rarely explicit in the studies we have reviewed, advocates can also provide more or less formal counselling and ongoing support. Therefore, we can locate advocates at the interface between two dimensions of care in the model depicted in Fig. 6.1: they engage with individual clients who are being abused, aiming to empower them and linking them to the wider context of community services. In some health settings they may also have a role in bringing about system change, catalysing increased recognition by clinicians of women experiencing abuse. In a pilot study for a primary care-based programme that two of us (GF and JR) are implementing, the domestic violence advocate, seconded by a voluntary domestic violence organization, is directly engaged in educating clinicians about direct inquiry and about appropriate responses to disclosure. She is also responsible for monitoring of the frequency of direct inquiry about abuse and referrals to advocacy.

On the whole, controlled studies of advocacy within health care settings have detected a reduction in rates of abuse or increased use of community resources by women, although most have weak study designs and small sample sizes.

The highest quality study of advocacy, with two-year follow-up of participants, is Sullivan's landmark trial[12] outside the context of health care. Women ($n = 282$) were recruited from shelters (refuges) in the mid-western United States and randomly allocated to intervention and control groups. Intervention participants met with women undergraduates who had received training in domestic violence advocacy. The intervention was intensive: 4–6 hours/week over a 10-week period, focusing on access to community resources: housing, employment, legal assistance, education, child care, transport, and social support. Participants in the intervention group experienced substantially less violence over time and reported higher quality of life, although not improved mental health status. Detailed analysis showed that obtaining community resources and increased social support were prerequisites for improved quality of life and reduced violence.[13] It would be misleading to generalize this study from the specific population of participants it recruited – women who had successfully left an abusive relationship and obtained community resources in the form of a shelter or refuge – to the broader population of women who disclose to clinicians. The latter group may still be in an abusive relationship and may be completely isolated. Moreover, the intensity of the advocacy intervention in this study, albeit from trained university student volunteers rather than domestic violence professionals, may be difficult to reproduce in mainstream domestic violence programmes.

Domestic violence advocates may also be effective in other contexts. A controlled trial from the criminal justice system of advocacy support to 81 women seeking temporary restraining orders found a reduction in physical and psychological abuse compared to women receiving standard court services.[14]

The largest controlled study of advocacy in a health care setting is Muelleman and colleagues'[15] comparison of outcomes for 222 women physically injured by partners before and after an advocacy service was implemented in an emergency department. The study found an increase in shelter use and in uptake of shelter-based counselling but no reduction in violence nor in emergency department visits.

Advocacy may be combined with other interventions. A controlled study of 288 pregnant Hispanic women by Parker and colleagues[16] in the United States compared women receiving counselling plus advocacy to those receiving just counselling, with a group receiving written information on resources acting as a control group. Two months after giving birth, women in all three groups experienced less violence, with a significant difference in reporting of violence between the counselling plus advocacy versus counselling alone groups. This is an important finding in a reasonably powered parallel group study with comparable groups, although there was the potential for contamination (i.e. women allocated to one group receiving part of the intervention from another group) between groups that would have reduced differences in effect size. Fanslow and colleagues' study of advocacy (including safety planning) and counselling in a New Zealand emergency department found an increase in referrals to outside agencies at three months[17] that was not sustained after a year.[18]

In spite of the small number and methodological limitations of relevant studies and the variation in advocacy models, there is evidence that advocacy can be an effective intervention for women experiencing partner abuse. This quantitative evidence is complemented by qualitative research.

One of us (MZ) has carried out a qualitative study of pregnant women who had received services after a partner violence intervention in primary care. The aim of the interviews was to understand what happens *after* the screening and disclosure phase with women who had received care from an advocate in a domestic violence intervention program in a family medicine setting in New York. Informants described vividly the helpfulness of approaches championed by community advocates: support, education, and advocacy. Survivors also reported the need for long-term care in most situations, whether for social services or ongoing support. They described success as feeling empowered and safer, while both in or out of the abusive relationship.

Clinician referral or self referral, after encouragement from a clinician or publicity about advocacy services in a health care setting, are both legitimate routes to advocacy support. It is our experience that formal referral with the woman's consent is more likely to result in advocacy involvement. It has the added advantage of being a familiar part of the clinician's repertoire: referral to other specialists or agencies is common in clinical, particularly primary care, practice. While we recognize the danger of reproducing the professional power of the medical model vis-à-vis a woman experiencing abuse, avoidance of direct referral may ultimately contribute to her continuing isolation and powerlessness.

PSYCHOLOGICAL INTERVENTIONS

The psychological interventions that have been evaluated are heterogeneous, and include counselling, feminist therapy, and use of cognitive behavioural models. The papers reporting these studies rarely have sufficient information to characterize or replicate the interventions. In his systematic review of psychosocial interventions, Abel[6] (p.13) concludes that little attention is given to describing 'either the specifics of the intervention or the theoretical framework(s) that supports it.' Within political movements that challenge domestic violence there is a strong critique of psychological interventions for women who are abused by their partners. This critique highlights the danger of reducing what is essentially an external problem to an internal psychological disorder that needs 'therapy'.[19]

Individual descriptions of the experience of abuse are replete with accounts of pejorative and degrading comments by the abusive partner, with frequent and repetitive insults about mental health problems that may or may not exist. In the acute phase of domestic violence, it is difficult to know whether depression, anxiety, sleep disturbance, and even paranoid behaviour are functional. The overlay of fear and suspicion that is the norm in the context of a relationship with unpredictable and ongoing danger can seem pathological to providers inexperienced in the treatment of domestic violence. These problems have created a potential for re-victimization by professionals, particularly within criminal justice and health care systems. Survivors are improperly diagnosed and treated, and judges may believe statements from the abusive partner, leading to dual arrests and inappropriate placement of children. Given this backdrop, psychological treatment for the sequelae of domestic violence is regarded with suspicion by some domestic violence activists. Nevertheless, there are a number of studies that have investigated the effect of psychological treatments for women experiencing partner abuse.

We have already mentioned Parker's study,[16] which showed no difference between unlimited counselling and giving women information about resources. Fanslow showed that there was a relatively short-lived effect on referral of women disclosing abuse after introduction of single contact counselling and advocacy programme in an emergency department.[18] A small Korean study (33 women), with a large loss to follow-up, showed no difference between a group intervention using a problem-solving/empowerment model and no intervention on most mental health outcomes.[19] An even smaller study (20 women) comparing the effects of feminist-oriented and grief-oriented counselling in women presenting for counselling in a battered women's programme found that only the latter improved self-esteem and self-efficacy.[20] An equally small (20 women) controlled study of a twice weekly cognitive behavioural programme over 20 weeks in Columbia showed a reduction in abuse.[21]

It is still unclear whether psychological interventions are effective for women who are still experiencing or have recently experienced intimate partner abuse (IPA). What is clear is that counselling on its own is not an adequate intervention and may increase a woman's sense of isolation and possibly her safety if it is not dovetailed with advocacy. Within the terms of our model, if psychological interventions work for women experiencing recent abuse, they do so at the individual level, with empowerment as a key component.

The lack of explicitness and standardization of models and techniques hampers research. This may conflict with a need for psychological interventions to be targeted more specifically at women in different stages of abusive relationships; for example distinguishing between women still living with an abusive partner and those who have left. As Abel[6] argues, we need more homogeneous treatment groups to minimize the confounding of the effect of psychological interventions.

In spite of insufficient research on outcomes of psychological interventions, there are several sources of guidance for psychologists or counsellors who have clients with recent experience of partner abuse. These range from Mary Ann Dutton's classic text, in which she articulates her empowerment model,[22] to Lenore Walker's generic guide to survivor therapy[23] and the more recent manual developed by Roxanne Agnew-Davies, targeted at mental health professionals working specifically with women experiencing or escaping domestic violence.[24]

Whatever model of treatment is used, the content of interventions needs to take into account women's risk for further violence even if they have left an abusive relationship. The overall goals for therapy, as articulated by Agnew-Davies, include:

- crisis intervention;
- dealing with psychological impact of abuse;
- shortening the time taken to regain a sense of well-being;
- preventing long-term damaging effects of abuse left unrecognized or unacknowledged.

The first session with women who have recently experienced abuse needs to prioritize external safety, confidentiality, appropriate pacing, being non-judgemental, and containment. Subsequent sessions should have a standard structure: establishing the therapeutic alliance, assessing needs and agreeing goals, active work, consolidation, and closure/future planning. These sessions can tackle specific topics such as flashbacks and intrusive memories, avoidance and numbing, anger, anxiety, depression, sleeping difficulties, and low self-esteem. Agnew-Davies argues that diagnostic categories for women who have *recently* experienced abuse are confounded by the psychological impact of abuse and are not needed for psychological interventions.

The potential for couple therapy is debatable. Dutton writes that she recommends it only when three conditions have been met: the threat of further abuse has been 'greatly reduced'; the abusive and controlling behaviour has ceased for a longer period than the longest lapse between previous episodes; both partners agree that they want to repair the damage to the relationship caused by the abuse. Agnew-Davies is more sceptical about couple counselling or family therapy in the context of a history of partner abuse, and cites evidence that it is not only ineffective but that it also increases the risk of harm to women.

SYSTEM CHANGE AND COMMUNITY-BASED RESPONSE

The evidence, as we have reviewed it above, is organized in terms of interventions, either individual or in combinations. We maintain that there is sufficient evidence to inform the initial response of health practitioners to women who disclose partner abuse and to recommend referral to specialist advocacy services and, possibly, some form of psychological intervention. But this conclusion belies the challenge of implementing changes in clinician behaviour, which requires system changes within the health care setting, and the obstacles in linking clinical to advocacy services. Implementation of these recommendations requires a cultural change in many clinical settings and organizational development in forging partnerships with agencies with expertise in IPA. This is not unique to responding to IPA; changes in management of chronic illness also require an implementation strategy.[25] Nevertheless, changing practice around IPA has added obstacles coming from attitudes of clinicians towards the issue, the substantial risk to the safety of women experiencing abuse, and the interface with the criminal justice system. Training of health care professionals to help them implement appropriate responses to abused women and provision of additional resources to support liaison with, and referral to, outside agencies are essential. Education of health care professionals is discussed in Chapter 4.

FIRST DO NO HARM

One of the limitations of research on interventions with women who have recently experienced IPA is the virtual silence about the potential harm arising from these interventions. Because of the history of domestic violence being invisible or marginalized as a problem by health care professionals (see Chapter 1), there has been an understandable implicit assumption on the part of many domestic violence advocates that *any* intervention within health services is better than none. But survivors are concerned about breaches of confidentiality and the potential for increased risk after disclosure. There is also a danger that the clinicians' uncertainty about how to respond to disclosure, and absence of knowledge about advocacy and access to community services, could leave the woman who has disclosed feeling more isolated and vulnerable. In the studies we have highlighted above, where interventions appear to benefit women, training of clinicians is central. Domestic violence is either absent or barely present in most medical and nursing school curricula in the UK and Australia, although it is gaining a foothold in North America.[26] This means that developing and implementing appropriate health service responses to IPA require systematic training of clinicians. There is some evidence about effective training, although this has largely been evaluated in terms of changes in attitudes and knowledge, which cannot be assumed to result in changes in clinician behaviour.[27]

GUIDELINES

We have not systematically searched for guidelines. Instead we have chosen national guidelines from four countries (UK,[28] Canada,[29] US,[30] and New Zealand[31]) that are freely available on websites. We have appraised these guidelines using a validated appraisal tool that addresses the quality of guideline development (i.e. the likelihood that they are based on the research evidence in a relatively unbiased way).[32] On the whole, the guidelines score poorly on appraisal, largely because their development methods are opaque and the link between evidence and recommendations not clear, with the exception of the Canadian guidelines, which are directly based on a systematic review. Moreover, the guidelines do differ in recommendations with regards to screening: the US and New Zealand guidelines recommending this unequivocally, the Canadian stating there is insufficient evidence to make a recommendation, and the UK advocating a low threshold for asking. The guidelines disagree to a lesser extent on actions following disclosure; notably, referral to advocacy or other expert agencies is absent from the UK guidelines and there is no mention of the importance of training in the UK or Canadian guidelines.

Below we present the main recommendations within these guidelines for management of IPA in health care settings. *Italicized text is quoted directly from the guidelines.* Other text is our summary.

Domestic violence: the general practitioner's role

(UK Royal College of General Practitioners 1998)
These are pragmatic, relatively brief guidelines focused on primary care.

1. Consider the possibility.

Be open to the signs that could indicate abuse: lists 17 possibilities, e.g. unexplained bruises, type of injury is inconsistent with explanation, patient has history of miscarriage.

2. Emphasize confidentiality.
3. Ask the question.

Not universally but with a very low threshold for suspected abuse.

4. Document.
5. Photographs.

When appropriate:

6. Assess present situation.
7. Provide information.
8. Devise a safety plan.

All of the above recommendations are fleshed out and four of the eight include references to specific studies (recommendations 1, 3, 4, 7).

Prevention and treatment of violence against women: systematic review and recommendations

(Canadian Task Force on Preventive Health Care, 2001. (And statement from the Canadian Task Force on Preventive Health Care: Wathen CN, MacMillan HL. CMAJ 2003; 169:582–584.))
These are strictly evidence-based guidelines and reflect the paucity of primary studies.

- *There is insufficient evidence to recommend for or against routine universal screening for violence against either pregnant or non-pregnant women (grade I recommendation); however, clinicians should be alert to the signs and symptoms of potential abuse and may wish to ask about exposure to abuse during diagnostic evaluation of these patients.*
- *There is insufficient evidence to recommend any of the following primary care interventions to prevent violence against pregnant or non-pregnant women,*

although decisions to do so may be made by the clinician and patient on other grounds:

- *primary care counselling (grade I recommendation)*
- *referral to shelters (grade I recommendation)*
- *referral to personal and vocational counselling (grade I recommendation)*

■ *There is fair evidence (level 1) to refer women who have spent at least 1 night in a shelter to a structured program of advocacy services (grade B recommendation).*

Graded recommendations go from A (good evidence to recommend) through to E (good evidence to recommend against), with Grade B recommendation meaning that there is fair evidence to recommend the clinical preventive action. An I recommendation means that there is insufficient evidence (in quantity and/or quality) to make a recommendation; however, other factors may influence decision-making. Level 1 evidence means that there is evidence from at least one randomized control trial.

National consensus guidelines on identifying and responding to domestic violence in health care settings

(Family Violence Prevention Fund, USA, September 2002)
We have summarized these extensive guidelines. They are uncritical of the small pool of research and its questionable quality. There is no linkage of recommendations to evidence.

Prerequisites

- Health care provider to have received appropriate education, with training on how to ask about violence and how to respond when it is identified.
- Health care provider to have developed site-specific policies.

Screening

- Health providers should screen patients for current and lifetime exposure to intimate partner violence victimization, including direct questions about physical, emotional, and sexual abuse (although it is recognized that asking about lifetime abuse may not be possible in some health care settings, such as the emergency room).
- All adolescent and adult patients (female and male), regardless of cultural background, should be screened, as should parents or caregivers of children in paediatric settings.
- Screening should be conducted routinely, regardless of the presence or absence of indicators of abuse. However, screening should not occur if the provider cannot:
  - Assure privacy/confidentiality (except for legal/ethical obligations to disclose).
  - Assure safety of the patient or provider.
  - Provide a professional interpreter if needed.
- Males should not be screened if extra precautions have not been put in place.

Interventions

For all patients who disclose abuse providers should:

- Provide validation.
- Provide information.
- Assess safety/health.
- Make referrals to local resources.
- Document.
- Follow-up with at least one appointment with health professional, social worker, or advocate.

Family violence intervention guidelines: child and partner abuse

(New Zealand Ministry of Health, 2002)
Similar to the family violence prevention fund guidelines. No critical appraisal of the evidence and no linkage between recommendations and evidence. Raises issue of potential harm by not screening and misdiagnosing, but says nothing about the risks related to screening. Sees screening as an intervention in itself. No mention of lack of evidence about the effectiveness of interventions post-identification.

Prerequisites

- Health care provider to have received appropriate training on how to ask about violence and how to respond when it is identified.
- Health care provider to have established working relationships and referral pathways with local agencies prior to undertaking intervention for family violence.
- All interviews with patients to take place in private and be confidential (except for legal/ethical obligations to disclose), with professional interpreters if needed.

The primary recommendation is for routine screening. This is based on an uncritical view of the evidence citing the following points:

- abuse is frequently missed in patient encounters with health professionals;
- case-finding and screening of high risks do not improve identification rates;
- early diagnosis has potential to improve outcomes, both as an intervention in its own right and as an avenue to accessing help from other organizations;
- brief screening tests are sensitive, specific, acceptable to women, and substantially improve detection;
- resource implications for implementing screening are not great.

See Chapter 5 for further discussion of the problematic nature of the evidence for screening women for domestic violence in health care settings.

The guidelines discuss a six-step model for identifying and responding to family violence within health care settings:

1. Identification using simple direct questions asked in a non-threatening manner.
   - Routinely screen all females aged 16 years and over (where frequency of screening differs as a function of health care setting and circumstances of the presentation; e.g. annually where there is an ongoing relationship between the patient and family physician and no suspicion of abuse, every visit to the ED).
   - Question all females aged 12–15 years presenting with signs and symptoms indicative of abuse.
   - Question all males aged 16 years and over presenting with signs and symptoms indicative of abuse.
2. Provision of emotional support.
3. Assessment of risk.
4. Safety planning and referral.
5. Documenting injuries.
6. Referral to specialist agencies, if required.

CONCLUSION

Despite the relative weakness of research evidence, it is possible to articulate an appropriate response for clinicians when faced with disclosure of IPA: immediate validation and emotional support, strict confidentiality, documentation, checking the safety of the woman and her children, ongoing support, and referral to expert services/advocacy. This core response needs to be supported by system change within the clinical setting and integrated within a coordinated community response to IPA.

Researchers always say that 'more research is needed' and we are no exception. But in the case of developing the management of IPA in health care settings, it is unarguable that more research will help. In particular, we require controlled studies of health care-based interventions that are reasonably powered to detect differences in women-centred outcomes, such as abuse, quality of life, and mental health measures. These need to be complemented by qualitative studies exploring in greater depth the priorities of women who have experienced IPA. We also require better research on interventions to tackle the long-term psychosocial sequelae of IPA. Broader policy research is needed to develop implementation models to integrate activity within clinical services with a wider, coordinated, community-based response, strengthening the status and funding of advocacy services.

Finally, there is a danger that the patchy evidence base for how clinicians should respond to IPA can be used as an excuse for health services not to do anything. We believe that this would be a gross distortion of the argument we have pursued in this chapter and that the general case is for a core response of clinicians, even if the details need further evidence.

REFERENCES

1. Bacchus L, Mezey G, Bewley S. Women's perceptions and experiences of routine enquiry for domestic violence in a maternity service. Brit J Obstet Gynaec 2002; 109:9–16.

2. Wathen CN, MacMillan HL. Interventions for violence against women: scientific review. JAMA 2003; 289:589–600.
3. Klevens J, Sadowski L. Women's health: intimate partner violence. Clin Evid 2003 [accessed 19/9/04]. Available from: http://www.clinicalevidence.com/ceweb/conditions/woh/1013/1013.jsp
4. Ramsay J, Richardson J, Carter YH, et al. Should health professionals screen women for domestic violence? Systematic review. BMJ 2002; 325:314.
5. Davidson LL, King V, Garcia J, et al. What role can the health services play? In: Taylor-Browne J, ed. What works in reducing domestic violence: a comprehensive guide for professionals. London: Whiting & Birch; 2001:95–122.
6. Abel EM. Psychosocial treatments for battered women: a review of empirical research. Res Soc Work Pract 2000; 10:55–77.
7. Taket A, Nurse J, Smith K, et al. Routinely asking women about domestic violence in health settings. BMJ 2003; 327:673–676.
8. Dienemann J, Campbell J, Landenburger K, et al. The domestic violence survivor assessment: a tool for counselling women in intimate partner violence relationships. Patient Educ Couns 2002; 46:221–228.
9. Dutton MA. Empowering and healing the battered woman. New York: Springer; 1992.
10. Gerbert B, Abercrombie P, Caspers N, et al. How health care providers help battered women: the survivor's perspective. Women Health 1999; 29:115–135.
11. Gerbert B, Caspers N, Bronstone A, et al. A qualitative analysis of how physicians with expertise in domestic violence approach the identification of victims. Ann Intern Med 1999; 131:578–584.
12. Sullivan CM, Bybee DI. Reducing violence using community-based advocacy for women with abusive partners. J Consult Clin Psychol 1999; 67:43–53.
13. Bybee DI, Sullivan CM. The process through which an advocacy intervention resulted in positive change for battered women over time. Am J Community Psychol 2002; 30:103–132.
14. Bell ME, Goodman LA. Supporting battered women involved with the court system: an evaluation of a law school-based advocacy intervention. Violence Against Women 2001; 7:1377–1404.
15. Muelleman RL, Feighny KM. Effects of an emergency department-based advocacy program for battered women on community resource utilization. Ann Emerg Med 1999; 33:62–66.
16. Parker B, McFarlane J, Soeken K, et al. Testing an intervention to prevent further abuse to pregnant women. Res Nurs Health 1999; 22:59–66.
17. Fanslow JL, Norton RN, Robinson EM, et al. Outcome evaluation of an emergency department protocol of care on partner abuse. Aust N Z J Public Health 1998; 22:598–603.
18. Fanslow JL, Norton RN, Robinson EM. One year follow-up of an emergency department protocol for abused women. Aust N Z J Public Health 1999; 23:418–420.
19. Kim S, Kim J. The effects of group intervention for battered women in Korea. Arch Psychiat Nurs 2001; 15:257–264.
20 Mancoske RJ, Standifer D, Cauley C. The effectiveness of brief counseling services for battered women. Res Soc Work Pract 1994; 4:53–63.
21. Laverde DI. Effects of cognitive-behavioural therapy in controlling wife abuse [in Spanish]. Revista de Analisis del Comportamieno 1987; 3:193–200.
22. Dutton MA. Empowering and healing the battered woman: a model for assessment and intervention. New York: Springer; 1992.
23. Walker LE. Abused women and survivor therapy: a practical guide for the psychotherapist. Washington, DC: American Psychological Association; 1994.
24. Agnew-Davies R. Manual for mental health professionals supporting women experiencing or escaping domestic violence. London: Refuge/Department of Health; 2004.
25. Grimshaw J, McAuley LM, Bero LA, et al. Systematic reviews of the effectiveness of quality improvement strategies and programmes. Qual Saf Health Care 2003; 12:298–303.
26. http://www.aamc.org/data/aib/cime/vo12no4.pdf [accessed 3/8/04].
27. Davidson LL, Grisso JA, Garcis-Moreno C, et al. Training programs for healthcare professionals in domestic violence. J Women Health Gend Based Med 2001; 10:953–969.

28. Heath I. Domestic violence: the general practitioner's role. London: Royal College of General Practitioners; 1998. Available from: http://www.rcgp.org.uk/rcgp/corporate/position/dom_violence/index.asp

29. Wathen CN, MacMillan HL. Prevention of violence against women. Recommendation statement from the Canadian Task Force on Preventive Health Care. Can Med Assoc J 2003; 169:582–584. Available from: http://www.ctfphc.org/Sections/Domestic_violence.htm

30. National consensus guidelines on identifying and responding to domestic violence in healthcare settings. Washington, DC: Family Violence Prevention Fund; 2002. Available from: http://endabuse.org/programs/healthcare/files/Consensus.pdf

31. Family violence intervention guidelines: child and partner abuse. Auckland: Ministry of Health; 2002. Available from: http://www.moh.govt.nz/moh.nsf

32. Cluzeau FA, Littlejohns P, Grimshaw JM, et al. Development and application of a generic methodology to assess the quality of clinical guidelines. Int J Qual Health Care 1999; 11:21–28. Available from: http://www.agreecollaboration.org/

Chapter 7

How is intimate partner abuse experienced by childbearing women?

Heather McCosker-Howard and Anne B Woods

Most time when it was like that, you had to get out a bit earlier because you knew what was in store. I think I used to put two in the pram and have the others walking. We used to go up to the hospital at all hours of the night for a few hours until it was safe to go home.

Sally, a survivor of intimate partner abuse

INTRODUCTION

The childbearing year, which extends from conception through pregnancy, birth, and the postpartum period, is typically a time of anticipation, adaptation, and growth. It is also a time of increased risk due to pregnancy-related conditions. Intimate partner abuse (IPA) is a serious risk during the childbearing year that endangers the health and life of pregnant women and their unborn children. Midwives, physicians, nurses, traditional birth attendants, and other health care providers in contact with pregnant and postpartum women are ideally situated to identify those who are currently abused or at risk for abuse by an intimate partner. This chapter will explore the prevalence of IPA during the childbearing year and review its impact on maternal, fetal, and neonatal health outcomes. To encourage a coordinated response between current research knowledge and maternity health care, suggestions for evidence-based clinical practice, teaching, and directions for research are provided.

PREVALENCE OF ABUSE DURING PREGNANCY

Abuse during pregnancy is more common than many other pregnancy-related complications, such as placenta preavia or pre-eclampsia.[1,2]

Among industrialized countries, the prevalence of IPA during pregnancy ranges from 0.9 to 20.1%, with the majority of studies reporting rates of 4–8%.[3–5] In developing countries, the prevalence is greater, with rates ranging from 4 to 32%.[3,6]

The wide range of prevalence estimates is influenced by numerous factors. Variations in IPA definitions among studies impact reported rates. The majority of studies define the concept of IPA in pregnancy as physical abuse, including being hit, shoved, slapped, kicked, being in a physical fight, or being physically hurt. The prevalence rates of only physical IPA in pregnancy range on the lower end of the spectrum, from 1.2 to 11%.[4,5] When sexual abuse is included in the definition, the prevalence of IPA in pregnancy increases to 16–33%.[7–10] Few studies include emotional or verbal abuse in the definition of IPA. A large, retrospective, multi-ethnic, multisite study of 1,004 women immediately postpartum found that 6–11% reported emotional abuse during the pregnancy.[11] The authors note that the overall prevalence of abuse may be low since Cuban American women and women with either Mexican American or Central American partners were less likely to report emotional abuse compared to Anglo-Americans. This variation in reporting abuse may be related to fear of deportation for undocumented immigrants or to variations in cultural norms and acculturation levels. Higher rates of emotional abuse in pregnancy are reported by others. O'Campo and colleagues' investigation of 358 low-income women found a disturbing level of abuse during pregnancy, with 65% reporting either verbal abuse or physical violence. Forty-five per cent experienced only negative verbal interaction and the major perpetrator was identified as the male partner.[12] Study participants were predominately young (69% under 24 years of age), poor, unmarried, African-American, and with less than a high school education – all factors associated with increased risk for IPA – which may account for the unusually high prevalence in this study. However, similar prevalence rates for emotional and verbal abuse in pregnancy were found in a sample of 475 pregnant women in Turkey (44.9%)[8] as well as among a sample of 207 married or cohabitating women (44.4%) visiting antenatal clinics in Sweden.[13] Multiple types of violence – physical, sexual, and emotional/verbal – frequently coexist in the scenario of IPA.

Differences in study methodology and sampling may also affect prevalence rates. In population-based studies, the prevalence of IPA in pregnancy is typically lower than in clinically based samples. Utilizing the Pregnancy Risk Assessment Monitoring System (PRAMS), data from 16 states in the US were analysed, with 64,994 respondents and representing 2,776,328 births. A prevalence rate of 4.1% for physical abuse by a husband or partner during pregnancy was found. If perpetrators in addition to the husband or partner were included, the prevalence rate rose to 5.3%.[14] Prevalence rates in clinically based samples typically range from 7 to 20%.[4] This difference may be explained by more limited questions about abuse in population-based data collection. The highest rates of IPA in pregnancy among clinically based samples were found when in-depth instruments were utilized, such as the Conflict Tactics Scale[15] or the Index of Spouse Abuse.[16] The age of study participants also impacts prevalence, with higher rates identified among pregnant adolescents compared to adult women. Parker and her colleagues found that 22% of pregnant teenagers reported abuse during pregnancy compared to 16% of adults in a sample of 691 women utilizing an urban prenatal clinic setting in the US.[17] Similarly high prevalence rates were found in an Australian multicentre study of 570 pregnant teenagers, aged 12–17 years, in which 157 (29.2%) reported IPA.[18] The developmental stage of adolescence affects variations in prevalence, with middle adolescents aged 16 to 17 years experiencing the highest rates compared to older adolescents.[19] The higher rates among pregnant adolescents are multifactorial and may be related to their inexperience with interpersonal relationships.

The timing of data collection during pregnancy has a substantial impact on IPA prevalence rates. Studies that interviewed women later in pregnancy, especially in the third trimester, or that asked more than once during the same pregnancy, identified higher reported rates of violence. In an Australian antenatal clinic study, 1,014 pregnant women were interviewed regarding their history of IPA. In the current pregnancy, 5.8% had experienced IPA, but this rate rose to 8.9% when women were interviewed at 36 weeks.[20] Parker and her colleagues found that 8% of women identified as non-abused at the first prenatal visit reported subsequent abuse during the second or third trimesters.[17]

The other important time during the childbearing year when women are at risk of experiencing IPA is the postpartum period. A survey of 2,648 participants from the North Carolina PRAMS found that 3.2% of women experienced postpartum abuse, with the majority of perpetrators being current or former husbands/partners.[21] The majority of women in this study (85%) were 20 years of age or older.

Another US study found that among 570 adolescents the prevalence of IPA was highest in the first three months (21%) postpartum.[22] Similar to findings of increased risk for IPA in pregnancy, teens may be at increased risk for IPA during the postpartum period. A previous history of abuse, either prior to or during the pregnancy, is a strong risk factor for postpartum abuse.

IPA during the childbearing year is prevalent, with up to one in five pregnant teens and one in six pregnant adult women reporting abuse.[17] In light of these rates, it is imperative to understand the patterns of violence and implications for maternal and neonatal health.

PATTERNS OF IPA DURING THE CHILDBEARING YEAR

The childbearing year is comprised of dynamic physical, emotional, and interpersonal change. The patterns of IPA may also change during pregnancy and postpartum. Although anecdotal evidence suggests that pregnancy may be a time of increased risk for IPA, there are conflicting findings in the research, with some studies showing no change in prevalence rates while others find either increased or diminished levels. Martin's research team found a similar prevalence of IPA among North Carolina women both before and during pregnancy with rates of 6.9% and 6.1%, respectively.[21] This pattern of similar IPA prevalence rates prior to (24.4%) and during pregnancy (24.6%) was also found in a sample of 914 pregnant women in Mexico.[23] In contrast to these findings, both Saltzman[14] and Goodwin[24] found a lower prevalence of physical abuse during pregnancy in an analysis of population-based data from PRAMS. Furthermore, Saltzman and her colleagues note that, compared to the year prior to pregnancy, the prevalence of IPA during pregnancy was lower even in women in the highest-risk categories: women of younger age, unmarried, having less than 12 years of education, unintended pregnancy, or stressful events experienced in the pregnancy.[14] A protective effect for pregnancy was also seen in a population-based study in Vancouver, British Columbia, in which IPA ceased during pregnancy for 31% of previously abused women.[25] Coker and her associates, in a cross-sectional survey of 755 women (1,862 pregnancies) attending family practice clinics in South Carolina, found that among women who experienced abuse during pregnancy nearly half reported that the abuse increased, while it remained the same for 26% and decreased in frequency for 25%.[26] These findings must be viewed cautiously, since the retrospective study design is subject to the risk of recall bias. The authors note that many of the women reported on pregnancies up to 20 years prior to the survey.

While pregnancy may be protective for some women, others report that violence began during the pregnancy. Forty per cent of Canadian women[27] and 18% of Australian women[28] reported that the first episode of IPA occurred in pregnancy. In population-based studies, a much lower proportion of women report the initiation of IPA during pregnancy (1–2%) or postpartum (1%).[14,21,25] The wide variation in initiation rates may be accounted for by differences in data collection, definitions of partner abuse, study samples, and a previous history of IPA.

A consistent finding in the literature, however, is that a history of IPA is a strong risk factor for abuse in the childbearing year, with 24–95% of women who report abuse during pregnancy also reporting abuse in the prior year.[14,17,21,24,25,29–31] Among women who experience IPA during pregnancy, the severity and frequency of abuse has also been found to increase.

In clinic samples, 4–49% report moderate to severe violence during pregnancy.[5,7,12,30] A recent investigation of 65 couples from two North Carolina prenatal clinics found that among women who reported IPA during pregnancy there was a statistically significant increase in the mean monthly frequency of psychological aggression (increase of 3.95 behaviours per month; $p < 0.01$) and sexual coercion (increase of 0.83 behaviours per month; $p = 0.04$) when they became pregnant. Physical assault rates, although a mean of 2.27 behaviours higher, were not statistically significant ($p = 0.81$).[31] Support for the findings of increased frequency and severity of IPA in pregnancy among women who are abused also comes from a study of 258 men convicted of spouse abuse in a treatment programme in New York. One in seven participants ($n = 33$) admitted perpetrating violence against a current partner while she was pregnant. As measured by the composite injury score, the frequency and severity scores were more than twice as high when women were pregnant then when not pregnant (M = 9.4 vs. 4.2, respectively; $p < 0.001$).[32]

Overall, it is estimated that approximately 25–50% of women who experience IPA find pregnancy to be a protective period, another 25% experience the same risk of abuse as prior to the pregnancy, and the remaining women may be at greater risk.[26,33] Among those who experience IPA in pregnancy, the frequency and severity of violence increases. This has serious implications for the health and life of the woman and her unborn child.

EFFECTS OF IPA DURING THE CHILDBEARING PERIOD

IPA has both direct and indirect effects on pregnancy outcomes. The actual physical trauma of IPA can directly affect the pregnancy, while indirect effects are comprised of behavioural or physiological responses that are associated with IPA. The following section will review pertinent literature related to IPA and selected pregnancy outcomes.

Physical trauma

As early as 1962, articles examining trauma and pregnancy outcomes in the USA identified physical abuse as a cause of fetal and maternal injury.[34] However, much of the early literature on trauma in pregnancy involves blunt abdominal trauma due to falls, motor vehicle accidents, and assaults, without differentiating IPA.[35,36] A recent, retrospective study of 476 cases of trauma in pregnancy was conducted in both a tertiary care centre and a community hospital in North Carolina. The researchers found that 22% of trauma cases in pregnancy were due to domestic abuse and assaults with most of these occurring before 18 weeks gestation.[37] However, less than one-third of women who are injured from IPA during the childbearing year receive medical attention for their injuries.[20,21]

Research focusing on fetal trauma related to IPA in pregnancy has consistently found negative health consequences for the unborn child. The direct effects of trauma on the fetus depend on the gestational age, the type, location, and severity of the trauma, and the extent of disruption to normal uterine and fetal physiology. The location of injury patterns in pregnant women are more likely to be central, including blows to the head, torso, abdomen, breasts, and genitalia.[30,38] Abuse directed at the abdomen may particularly lead to poor pregnancy outcomes and perinatal death due to placental abruption, maternal uterine rupture, antepartal haemorrhage, and premature rupture of membranes.[5,37–39] The association of partner abuse and perinatal death is also found in developing countries. A community survey of 1,842 women in India found that even after adjusting for other confounders the odds of fetal and infant death are significantly greater for women who are abused by their husbands compared to non-abused women.[40]

Conflicting results in the literature are found for miscarriage, or spontaneous abortion, associated with IPA. Coker and her colleagues found that women abused during pregnancy had twice the risk of perinatal death, but not miscarriage, compared to non-abused women.[26] Other researchers have found that women who experience any type of IPA are significantly more likely to miscarry.[41,42] It is possible that physical or sexual trauma from IPA could result in early pregnancy loss, but there are multiple factors that can also account for pregnancy loss prior to 20 weeks gestation, including maternal endocrine imbalance, immunological factors, infections, systemic disorders, anomalies of the reproductive tract, and chromosomal abnormalities in the products of conception. Further research is warranted to identify the role and mechanisms of IPA in early pregnancy loss.

There is a growing recognition that the most severe trauma outcome of abuse in pregnancy is pregnancy-related maternal homicide. In an examination of 651 autopsy reports in Washington, DC, the second most common cause of death among pregnant women was intentional trauma, although rates of IPA are not provided.[43] However, Campbell and her colleagues, in an 11-city study of risk factors for femicide in abusive relationships, found that 70% of the 307 femicide cases were physically abused prior to their deaths by the same intimate partner who killed them. Furthermore, the researchers point out that stalking, forced sex, and abuse during pregnancy represented strong risk factors for women being murdered by their partner in an abusive relationship.[44]

Pregnancy intention

Pregnancy intention relates to questions about whether or not the pregnancy was planned and who or what influenced the decision to continue the pregnancy. Unintended pregnancy is most frequently defined as an unwanted or mistimed pregnancy. Women with unintended pregnancies have 2.4–4 times greater risk of experiencing physical abuse compared to women with intended pregnancies.[14,24] A small study ($n = 51$) of women presenting for abortion services at a clinic in North Carolina found that 22% reported current, past-year partner abuse.[45] In a larger study of 468 women over 18 years of age seeking abortions at an urban US abortion outpatient clinic, women were asked about any physical abuse over the previous year and/or any inflicted in the current pregnancy.[46] The timing of the pregnancy was the most common reason for termination in both abused and non-abused groups. However, abused women were significantly less likely to inform their partners of the pregnancy, to have their partners support the decision to abort, or to involve them in the process. Relationship issues significantly affected the abused women's decisions to abort, more so than those of the non-abused women. In trying to better understand the relationship between IPA and pregnancy intendedness, Campbell and her colleagues conducted focus groups in two geographically distinct domestic violence shelters. The connection between IPA and unintended pregnancy was through the partner's control of contraception and pressure from the partner to have a child.[47] The studies linking partner abuse, pregnancy intendedness, and abortions have limitations and the true prevalence of abuse among women seeking terminations requires more study.

Low birthweight

Low birthweight (LBW), defined as a weight less than 2,500 grams at birth, is associated with serious health problems for newborns, increased risk of long-term disabilities, and is a factor in 65% of infant deaths.[48] The aetiology of LBW is multifaceted and complex. Maternal behaviours, such as smoking, substance use, poor nutrition, late entry into prenatal care, close interpregnancy interval, and inadequate weight gain in pregnancy may account for LBW babies. Maternal medical problems, particularly essential chronic hypertension and infections, can affect birthweight. Likewise, pregnancy-related factors such as pregnancy-induced hypertension, multiple gestation, fetal defects, placental problems, intrauterine growth restriction, and preterm birth also impact birthweight.[49]

The role of IPA in pregnancy as a factor in LBW has been an area of intense interest. Initial studies consistently found significant associations of IPA and LBW. Battered women had a four-fold risk of delivering a LBW baby[50] and newborns of women who were abused in pregnancy weighed 133 grams less compared to newborns of non-abused women.[51] Unfortunately, early studies did not adjust for maternal behaviours or obstetric factors, which could mediate the relationship between IPA and LBW. A recent meta-analysis of eight studies found that women who experienced physical, sexual, or emotional abuse in pregnancy were 1.4 times more likely to give birth to a LBW baby than non-abused women.[52] However, after adjusting for potential confounders, the relationship between IPA and LBW was no longer statistically significant in these studies. In the most comprehensive investigation of IPA and birthweight, Kearney and her associates tested the mediation effect of negative maternal behaviours and social demographics while controlling for obstetric covariates in a sample of 1,969 women. Decreased birthweights were only found for single marital status (94 grams), smoking (97 grams), and low weight gain in pregnancy (187 grams). The effect of recent IPA in pregnancy on birthweight was explained by social and behavioural risk factors.[53] Each of these risk factors, however, may be viewed as an indirect effect of IPA. Substantial research has found significant associations of partner abuse in pregnancy and multiple negative maternal health behaviours and conditions that may impact pregnancy outcomes, including increased smoking and/or alcohol use,[30,54–57] delayed entry into prenatal care,[57,58] inconsistent prenatal care,[29] poor prenatal weight gain,[9] sexually transmitted infections and Group B Streptococcus in pregnancy,[59,60] and short intervals between pregnancies.[9,42]

Other factors may also affect the occurrence of LBW in women abused in pregnancy. Preterm birth, a factor associated with LBW, occurs significantly more often in women who report abuse during pregnancy. In a large clinic-based sample ($n = 401$) in the US, women who experienced severe IPA in pregnancy had 4.1 times greater risk of preterm labour (PTL) than non-abused women.[61] A dose–response relationship was also seen, with increasing severity of violence associated with increased incidence of PTL. Coker and her colleagues also found a dose–response relationship with increasing frequency of abuse during pregnancy and increased risk of preterm LBW deliveries (adjusted relative risk (RR) = 3.9; $p = 0.0004$).[26] The finding of a dose–response relationship, while not causal, does strengthen the support for an association of IPA in pregnancy with PTL and LBW.

Another mechanism through which IPA in pregnancy may impact LBW is stress. Among 808 low-income women, physical abuse was not associated with LBW after adjusting for other risk factors, but women who reported stress because of the abuse had 2.1 times greater odds of having a LBW infant, and the mean birthweight was 236 grams less compared to women who reported no stress because of abuse.[62] Other research found significantly greater stress among women who experience IPA in pregnancy compared to non-abused women.[55] There are biologically plausible pathways by which psychosocial stress may mediate the risk of preterm birth and LBW, but more research is needed in this area.

Postpartum depression

Adverse maternal postpartum outcomes are also associated with IPA.

While many women may have mild depressive symptoms, or 'baby blues' after birth, postpartum depression is intense and more persistent than postpartum blues, and has substantial effects on maternal–infant interactions and functional ability. In a small Canadian study of 30 women who reported abuse in pregnancy, 95% were abused in the first three months postpartum and 83% met diagnostic criteria for current psychiatric disorders, primarily major depressive disorder.[63] Larger studies were included in a recent systematic review of 18 articles that found fair evidence of a significant association between postpartum depression and partner abuse.[64] Postpartum depression was also associated with poor marital adjustment, recent stressful life events, lack of social support, and past psychiatric morbidity – all of which are prevalent in women who experience IPA. Additional risk factors for postpartum depression may also be found in abused women, such as low self-esteem, single marital status, low socioeconomic status, and unplanned pregnancy.

In developing countries, other risk factors may affect postpartum depression. In a prospective, longitudinal study in India, Patel and colleagues found that among 252 mothers interviewed 6–8 weeks postpartum 23% had postnatal depression. The prevalence remained almost identical (22%) for the 235 women who were interviewed again at six months postpartum. Similar to findings in developed countries, a history of antenatal psychiatric disorder was significantly associated with postnatal depression. But the risk of postpartum depression in women who experienced partner violence was significantly greater if the baby was a female (RR = 3.3).[65]

The aetiology of postpartum depression is complex and multifactorial. Women who experience IPA may be especially prone to the development of depressive disorder in the postpartum period due to multiple risk factors that are entwined within the abusive relationship.

Experiencing IPA during the childbearing year is associated with serious morbidity and mortality, for both the woman and her infant. In the era of evidence-based practice, it is important to understand what research suggests are the most effective and appropriate interventions to assist women to minimize the impact of abuse during the childbearing year.

INTERVENTIONS DURING THE CHILDBEARING YEAR

For many women, pregnancy serves as a point of entry into the health care system. Health care professionals who have contact with women during the childbearing year are uniquely poised to screen for IPA and initiate intervention. The first step in this process is identification of women who are abused or at risk for abuse by an intimate partner.

Identification and screening

For the purposes of identification there is inconsistent research to support clear predictors of IPA in pregnancy; however, some factors are certainly suggestive that a woman's circumstances warrant further investigation. In the above discussion on the effects of IPA in pregnancy, multiple direct and indirect factors were identified that could increase suspicion for IPA risk. These include evidence of physical trauma, increased smoking and/or alcohol use, delayed entry to, and inconsistent use of prenatal care, poor prenatal weight gain, sexually transmitted infections and Group B Streptococcus in pregnancy, short intervals between pregnancies, preterm labour and birth, and depressive symptoms. To further investigate predictors of IPA in pregnancy, a recent prospective study of 439 ethnically diverse women aged between 20 and 34 years from four public and private prenatal clinics in Alabama was undertaken. A total of 48 women reported IPA during the current pregnancy. In multivariate analyses, the best predictors were depression (adjusted odds ratio (AOR) = 2.5; $p < 0.001$), more stressful life events (AOR = 1.6; $p < 0.001$), lack of contraceptive use (AOR = 4.6; $p < 0.05$), and a lack of faith in God or a higher power (AOR = 3.4; $p < 0.05$).[29] Although this research requires replication with larger samples of women who report IPA during a current pregnancy, including teenagers, the findings may help alert health care providers to increase awareness for potential risk for IPA in pregnancy.

Special mention is warranted regarding late presentation or inadequate use of prenatal care. The attitude and responses of health professionals can be crucial in facilitating identification of IPA. If the response is negative and judgemental a woman may not disclose the reason for the delay: a missed opportunity for identification of a woman experiencing IPA.

There is increasing evidence supporting the use of routine assessment for abuse during pregnancy. Research suggests that women, even those who are not in an abusive relationship, believe it is important to ask about the possible presence of abuse.[66] Since a history of IPA is a strong risk factor for IPA in pregnancy, screening for past IPA may be of value. Due to the dynamic and fluctuating nature of IPA during the childbearing year, it is also imperative that screening be repetitive, occurring at least once each trimester as well as postpartum. Furthermore, because of the association of significantly increased risk for femicide when women are abused during pregnancy,[43,44] Campbell notes that universal assessment and intervention during pregnancy is vital to minimize the risk of death.[67] More in-depth discussion on some of the problems with screening practices is found in Chapter 5.

Referral, counselling, and support

Referral and the provision of support and information about services available for women who are experiencing abuse have been reported as important interventions.[68] In one small interview study of 16 women with children being visited by health visitors in the UK, difficulties in seeking help were clearly described.[69] Those who disclosed their experience of IPA did not perceive that they had always received appropriate support or protection, and information about accessing specialist services. These results point to the need for high-quality studies to identify best practices for intervention.

Parker and her colleagues tested an intervention in an ethnically stratified cohort of 199 pregnant women who had been abused by an intimate partner in the past year and were still in a relationship with the abuser.[70] Women in the intervention group ($n = 132$) received information on the cycle of violence, a danger assessment, available options, safety planning, and resource referrals. A comparison group of 67 women received wallet-sized cards listing community resources for IPA. At 6 months and 12 months post-delivery, women in the intervention group had significantly less physical and non-physical partner violence, even after adjusting for ethnicity and age. Further analysis of this same sample found that pregnant women who were in the intervention group had significantly increased use of safety behaviours, including hiding money or keys, asking a neighbour to call police, gathering important papers, and removing weapons from the home.[71]

An alternative approach tested by McFarlane and Wiist consisted of a community outreach programme that used an advocacy model of weekly social support, education, and assisted referrals for pregnant women.[72] The intervention was designed to assist women to access resources needed to prevent future abuse and promote a healthy pregnancy. Women were identified as experiencing abuse during routine screening at the first antenatal visit and advocacy was offered by 'mentor mothers' in the women's homes. Mentor mothers made 922 contacts with 100 women, 74% of which were by phone, and 870 referrals for medical and social services, abuse counselling, and other needs. The average number of referrals was 8.6 per woman. Pregnancy outcomes were not discussed in this article. The major limitation of the intervention appeared to be the time required and difficulties in maintaining regular contact with the women: advocates were successful in contacting the abused women only 33% of the time either by phone, home visit, or other meeting.

Another evaluation by McFarlane and colleagues compared three interventions – Brief, Counselling, and Outreach – during the antenatal period among a sample of 329 pregnant, physically abused Hispanic women.[73] Follow-up interviews were conducted at 2, 6, 12, and 18 months postpartum. The Brief intervention involved providing written resource material about safety and local community resources during their pregnancy and no further contact until 2 months postpartum. The Counselling intervention consisted of unlimited access to a bilingual professional counsellor throughout their pregnancy. The counsellor was available both face-to-face and via phone, with or without an appointment. The Outreach intervention consisted of unlimited counselling support and the use of a 'mentor mother'. There were no significant differences in resource use among the three different groups, and the severity of abuse decreased significantly for all groups at 6, 12, and 18 months ($p < 0.001$).

These studies provide needed information for health care providers to plan intervention once IPA is identified during pregnancy. Providing specific information about IPA, danger assessment, reviewing options, safety planning, and resources were shown to be as effective as more time-consuming interventions, such as community outreach and counselling. However, the use of lay outreach workers for pregnant women who experience IPA during the childbearing year merits additional study. The increased adoption of safety behaviours and significant decrease in physical abuse lends support to the value of incorporating safety planning information in routine prenatal care visits. The type of questions that might be included in a safety assessment are listed in Box 7.1.

Box 7.1 Safety behaviour questions based on the work of McFarlane et al.[73]

Have you ever:

- Hidden money?
- Hidden an extra set of house/car keys?
- Established a danger code with family members?
- Asked a neighbour to notify police under certain circumstances, e.g when violence begins/you fail to do certain things?
- Removed weapons?

Do you have available/hidden in a safe place:

- Your Medicare number/social security number?
- Identification such as passport/driver's licence (or a copy of the same)?
- Bank account numbers/extra bank account?
- Birth and marriage certificates (you and children)?
- Important phone numbers?
- Hidden bag with extra clothes (you and children)?

CONCLUSION

Violence against pregnant and postpartum women is a significant global public health problem, with up to one in six pregnant adult women, one in five pregnant adolescents, and one in five postpartum women experiencing abuse by an intimate partner. Multiple types of violence – physical, sexual, and emotional/verbal – coexist in the scenario of IPA during pregnancy. While the frequency of IPA may decrease for up to half of women during pregnancy, the remaining 50% find that violence remains the same or increases. For those who experience IPA in pregnancy, the severity of violence often increases.

The effects of IPA on pregnancy outcome may occur through direct and indirect mechanisms. Trauma due to physical abuse is associated with increased fetal, neonatal, and maternal morbidity and mortality. There are conflicting findings regarding the association of miscarriage with IPA, and further research is needed to identify potential mechanisms. A consistent finding in the literature is that women who experience unintended pregnancy are at greater risk for IPA in pregnancy. The most severe trauma outcome for women is pregnancy-related maternal homicide.

The association of LBW babies among women who experience IPA in pregnancy is mediated through social and behavioural risk factors, such as smoking and inadequate maternal weight gain. However, these negative maternal health behaviours are significantly associated with IPA. Any efforts to improve maternal health behaviours must be accompanied by IPA identification and intervention.

While potential prenatal predictors of IPA may help increase suspicion to facilitate identification in the clinical setting, the strongest risk factor for IPA in pregnancy is a history of partner abuse. Combined with the dynamic nature of abuse in pregnancy, this argues for routine, repeated assessment for IPA during the childbearing year. Once identified, even basic interventions such as providing information on safety planning and resources can have significant beneficial effects in decreasing violence.

Ongoing education and training is required for health professionals providing maternity care to ensure that IPA is recognized and systematically responded to as a significant health issue during pregnancy and the postpartum period. Further research is necessary to evaluate the effectiveness of interventions on maternal, fetal, and neonatal outcomes.

REFERENCES

1. Campbell JC, Woods AB, Chouaf KL, et al. Reproductive health consequences of intimate partner violence. Clin Nurs Res 2000; 9(3):217–237.
2. Gabbe SG, Niebyl JR, Simpson JL, eds. Obstetrics: normal and problem pregnancies, 4th edn. New York: Churchill Livingstone; 2001.
3. Campbell JC, Garcia de la Cadena C, Sharps PW. Abuse during pregnancy in industrialized and developing countries. Violence Against Women 2004; 10(7):770–789.
4. Gazmararian JA, Lazorick S, Spitz AM, et al. Prevalence of violence against pregnant women. JAMA 1996; 275(24):1915–1920.
5. Jasinski JL. Pregnancy and domestic violence: a review of the literature. Trauma Violence Abuse 2004; 5(1):47–64.

6. Nasir K, Hyder AA. Violence against pregnant women in developing countries. Eur J Public Health 2003; 13(2):105–107.

7. Hedin LW, Grimstad H, Moller A, et al. Prevalence of physical and sexual abuse before and during pregnancy among Swedish couples. Acta Obstet Gynecol Scand 1999; 78(4):310–315.

8. Sahin HA, Sahin HG. An unaddressed issue: domestic violence and unplanned pregnancies among pregnant women in Turkey. Eur J Contracept Reprod Health Care 2003; 8(2):93–98.

9. Parker B, McFarlane, J, Soeken K. Abuse during pregnancy: effects on maternal complications and birth weight in adult and teenage women. Obstet Gynecol 1994; 84:323–32.

10. Smikle CB, Sorem KA, Stain AJ, et al. Physical and sexual abuse in a middle-class obstetric population. South Med J 1996; 89(10):983–988.

11. Torres S, Campbell J, Campbell DW, et al. Abuse during and before pregnancy: prevalence and cultural correlates. Violence Vict 2000; 15(3):303–321.

12. O'Campo P, Gielen AC, Faden RR, et al. Verbal abuse and physical violence among a cohort of low-income pregnant women. Womens Health Issues 1994; 4(1):29–37.

13. Hedin LW, Janson PO. The invisible wounds: the occurrence of psychological abuse and anxiety compared with previous experience of physical abuse during the childbearing year. J Psychosom Obstet Gynaecol 1999; 20(3):136–144.

14. Saltzman LE, Johnson CHY, Gilbert BC, Goodwin MM. Physical abuse around the time of pregnancy: an examination of prevalence and risk factors in 16 states. Matern Child Health J 2003; 7(1):31–43.

15. Straus MA. Measuring interfamily conflict and violence: the Conflict tactics (CTS) Scale. J Marriage Fam 1979; 41:75–88.

16. Hudson WW, McIntosh SR. The assessment of spouse abuse: two quantifiable dimensions. J Marriage Fam 1981:873–885.

17. Parker B, McFarlane J, Soeken K, et al. Physical and emotional abuse in pregnancy: a comparison of adult and teenage women. Nurs Res 1993; 42(3):173–178.

18. Quinlivan J, Evans, S. A prospective cohort study of the impact of domestic violence on young teenage pregnancy outcomes. J Pediatr Adolesc Gynecol 2001; 14: 17–23.

19. Curry MA, Doyle BA, Gilhooley J. Abuse among pregnant adolescents: differences by developmental age. MCN Am J Matern Child Nurs 1998; 23(3):144–150.

20. Webster J, Sweett S, Stolz TA. Domestic violence in pregnancy: a prevalence study. Med J Aust 1994; 161(8):466–470.

21. Martin SL, Mackie L, Kupper LL, et al. Physical abuse of women before, during, and after pregnancy. JAMA 2001; 285(12):1581–1584.

22. Harrykissoon SD, Rickert VI, Wiemann CM. Prevalence and patterns of intimate partner violence among adolescent mothers during the postpartum period. Arch Pediat Adol Med 2002; 156(April):325–330.

23. Castro R, Peek-Asa C, Ruiz A. Violence against women in Mexico: a study of abuse before and during pregnancy. Am J Public Health 2003; 93(7):1110–1116.

24. Goodwin MM, Gazmararian JA, Johnson CH, et al. PRAMS Working Group. Pregnancy intendedness and physical abuse around the time of pregnancy: findings form the Pregnancy Risk Assessment Monitoring System, 1996–1997. Matern Child Health J 2000; 4(2):85–92.

25. Janssen PA, Holt VL, Sugg NK, et al. Intimate partner violence and adverse pregnancy outcomes: a population-based study. Am J Obstet Gynecol 2003; 188(5):1341–1347.

26. Coker AL, Sanderson M, Dong B. Partner violence during pregnancy and risk of adverse pregnancy outcomes. Paediatr Perinat Epidemiol 2004; 18:260–269.

27. British Columbia Reproductive Care Program, 2003. Available from: http://www.rcp.gov.bc.ca

28. Taft A. Violence against women in pregnancy and after childbirth: current knowledge and issues in health care responses. Australian Domestic & Family Violence Clearinghouse; Issues Paper 6, 2002.

29. Dunn LL, Oths KS. Prenatal predictors of intimate partner abuse. J Obstet Gynecol Neonatal Nurs 2004; 33(1):54–63.

30. Hedin LW, Janson PO. Domestic violence during pregnancy: the prevalence of physical injuries, substance use, abortions and miscarriages. Acta Obstet Gynecol Scand 2000; 79(8):625–630.

31. Martin SL, Harris-Britt A, Li Y, et al. Changes in intimate partner violence during pregnancy. J Fam Violence 2004; 19(4):201–210.

32. Burch RL, Gallup GG. Pregnancy as a stimulus for domestic violence. J Fam Violence 2004; 19(4):243–247.

33. Campbell JC, Oliver CE, Bullock LFC. The dynamics of battering during pregnancy: women's explanations of why. In: Campbell JC, ed. Empowering survivors of abuse: health care for battered women and their children. Thousand Oaks, CA: Sage; 1998:81–89.

34. Dyer I, Barclay DL. Accidental trauma complicating pregnancy and delivery. Am J Obstet Gynecol 1962; 83:907–929.

35. Haycock CE. Blunt trauma in pregnancy. In: Haycock C, ed. Trauma and pregnancy. Littleton, MA: PSG; 1985:34–43.

36. Esposito RJ, Gens DR, Smith LG, et al. Evaluation of blunt abdominal trauma occurring during pregnancy. J Traum 1989; 29(12):1628–1632.

37. Connolly A, Katz VL, Bash KL, et al. Trauma and pregnancy. Am J Perinat 1997; 14(6):331–336.

38. Furniss KK. Violence against women. In: Lowdermilk DL, Perry SE, eds. Maternity and women's health care, 8th edn. St. Louis: Mosby; 2004:131–154.

39. Rachana C, Suraiya K, Hisha A. Prevalence and complications of physical violence during pregnancy. Eur J Obstet Gynecol Reprod Biol 2002; 103:26–29.

40. Jejeebhoy SJ. Associations between wife-beating and fetal and infant death: impressions from a survey in rural India. Stud Family Plann 1998; 29(3):300–308.

41. Renker PR. Physical abuse, social support, self-care, and pregnancy outcomes of older adolescents. J Obstet Gynecol Neonatal Nurs 1999; 28:377–388.

42. Jacoby M, Goenflo D, Black E, et al. Rapid repeat pregnancy and experiences of interpersonal violence among low-income adolescents. Am J Prev Med 1999; 16(4):318–321.

43. Krulewitch CJ, Pierre-Louis ML, de Leon-Gomez R, et al. Hidden from view: violent deaths among pregnant women in the District of Columbia, 1988–1996. J Midwifery Womens Health 2001; 46(1):4–10.

44. Campbell JC, Webster D, Koziol-McLain J, et al. Risk factors for femicide in abusive relationships: results from a multi-site case control study. Am J Public Health 2003; 93(7):1089–1097.

45. Evins G, Chescheir N. Prevalence of domestic violence among women seeking abortion services. Womens Health Issues 1996; 6(4):204–210.

46. Glander SS, Moore ML, Michielutte R, et al. The prevalence of domestic violence among women seeking abortion. Obstet Gynecol 1998; 91:1002–1006.

47. Campbell JC, Pugh LC, Campbell D, et al. The influence of abuse on pregnancy intention. Womens Health Issues 1995; 5(4):214–222.

48. March of Dimes Birth Defects Foundation. Quick reference: low birthweight. 2003; 09–285–0.

49. Piotrowshi KA. Labor and birth complications. In: Lowdermilk DL, Perry SE, eds. Maternity and women's health care, 8th edn. St. Louis: Mosby; 2004:983–1035.

50. McFarlane J. Battering during pregnancy: tip of an iceberg revealed. Women Health 1989; 15(3):69–84.

51. McFarlane J, Parker B, Soeken K. Abuse during pregnancy: associations with maternal health and infant birth weight. Nurs Res 1996; 45(1):37–42.

52. Murphy CC, Schei B, Myhr TL, et al. Abuse: a risk factor for low birth weight? A systematic review and meta-analysis. Can Med Assoc J 2001; 164(11):1567–1579.

53. Kearney MH, Munro BH, Kelly U, Hawkins J. Health behaviors as mediators for the effect of partner abuse on infant birthweight. Nurs Res 2004; 53(1):36–45.

54. Bullock LFC, Mears JCL, Woodcock C, et al. Retrospective study of the association of stress and smoking during pregnancy in rural women. Addict Behav 2000; 25:1–9.

55. Curry MA. The interrelationships between abuse, substance use, and psychosocial stress during pregnancy. J Obstet Gynecol Neonatal Nurs 1998; 27(6):692–699.

56. Grimstad H, Backe B, Jacobsen G, et al. Abuse history and health risk behaviors in pregnancy. Acta Obstet Gynecol Scand 1998; 77:893–897.
57. Webster J, Chandler J, Battistutta D. Pregnancy outcomes and health care use: effects of abuse. Am J Obstet Gynecol 1996; 174:760–767.
58. Dietz P, Gazmararian JA, Goodwin J, et al. Delayed entry into prenatal care: effect of physical violence. Obstet Gynecol 1997; 90(2):221–224.
59. Winn N, Records K, Rice, M. The relationship between abuse, sexually transmitted diseases and Group B Streptococcus in childbearing women. MCN Am J Matern Child Nurs 2003; 28(2):106–110.
60. Martin SL, Matza LS, Kupper LL, et al. Domestic violence and sexually transmitted diseases: the experience of prenatal care patients. Public Health Rep 1999; 114(3):262–268.
61. Shumway J, O'Campo P, Gielen A, et al. Preterm labor, placental abruption, and premature rupture of membranes in relation to maternal violence or verbal abuse. J Matern Fetal Med 1999; 8(3):76–80.
62. Altarac M, Strobino D. Abuse during pregnancy and stress because of abuse during pregnancy and birthweight. J Am Med Womens Assoc 2002; 57(4):208–214.
63. Stewart DE. Incidence of postpartum abuse in women with a history of abuse during pregnancy. Can Med Assoc J 1994; 151(11):1601–1604.
64. Wilson LM, Reid AJ, Midmer DK, et al. Antenatal psychosocial risk factors associated with adverse postpartum family outcomes. Can Med Assoc J 1996; 154(6):785–799.
65. Patel V, Rodrigues M, DeSouza N. Gender, poverty, and postnatal depression: a study of mothers in Goa, India. Am J Psychiatry 2002; 159(1):43–47.
66. Gielen AC, O'Campo PJ, Campbell JC, et al. Women's opinions about domestic violence screening and mandatory reporting. Am J Prev Med 2000; 19(4):279–285.
67. McFarlane J, Campbell JC, Sharps P, et al. Abuse during pregnancy and femicide: urgent implications for women's health. Obstet Gynecol 2002; 100(1):27–36.
68. Family Violence Prevention Fund. Preventing domestic violence: clinical guidelines on routine screening; 1999:23.
69. Peckover S. 'I could have just done with a little more help': an analysis of women's help-seeking from health visitors in the context of domestic violence. Health Soc Care Community 2003; 11(3):8.
70. Parker B, McFarlane J, Soeken K, et al. Testing an intervention to prevent further abuse to pregnant women. Res Nurs Health 1999; 22(1):59–66.
71. McFarlane J, Parker B, Soeken K, et al. Safety behaviours of abused women after an intervention during pregnancy. J Obstet Gynecol Neonatal Nurs 1998; 27(1):64–69.
72. McFarlane J, Wiist WH. Preventing abuse to pregnant women: implementation of a 'mentor mother' advocacy model. J Commun Health Nurs 1997; 14(4):237–249.
73. McFarlane J, Soeken K, Wiist W. An evaluation of interventions to decrease intimate partner violence to pregnant women. Public Health Nurs 2000; 17(6):443–451.

Chapter 8

What is the impact of intimate partner abuse on children?

Jennifer Smith

When the violence started my child cried and screamed, 'Don't hit Mummy. I hate you'. He tried to protect me and would cuddle me.

My child was very protective towards me. She would hit and yell at her father and tell him to stop. She would cuddle and comfort her younger sister.

Gail and Sue, mothers of young children

CHAPTER CONTENTS

INTRODUCTION

Intimate partner abuse (IPA) is not an 'adults only' problem. Research indicates that living in a family where a parent is being abused is a disturbing experience for children that can have negative effects on their emotional, behavioural, social, and cognitive development as well as their physical and mental health.[1-7] This chapter discusses the effects of IPA on children and the health professionals' role in the identification, assessment, and treatment of children living in abusive homes. In the introductory section children's direct and indirect experiences of IPA and the prevalence of this problem are discussed. The second section summarizes research findings about the relationship between exposure to IPA and children's short-term and long-term adjustment. Section three discusses a number of child and family factors which may exacerbate or attenuate the impact of IPA on children's well-being. The final section provides an overview of issues relating to identification, assessment and therapeutic intervention with children exposed to IPA.

DEFINING CHILDREN'S EXPERIENCES OF IPA

The early literature on IPA referred to children as 'silent victims' or 'witnesses' of abuse.[8,9] Today, they are more frequently described as 'children exposed to IPA' as the term 'exposure' is more inclusive of the complex diversity of overt, subtle, and sometimes hidden abusive behaviours that impact on children.[10] Other preferred definitions have included children 'experiencing', 'affected by', or 'living with' IPA as these terms emphasize that it affects children's lives in many ways.[1,11]

The predicament of children who are living with IPA may include a wide range of experiences. Many children may directly witness IPA and some will be all the more terrified because the abuse is occurring to one of the most significant adults in their lives. Sometimes children overhear what is happening and the abuse may be magnified or diminished in their imagination as a result of not seeing the actual events.[1,2] Other children will physically intervene in IPA to protect their parent and some may even become the victim of physical abuse themselves.[12-15] Children can also be exposed to the results of IPA without either hearing or seeing the acts of abuse. For example, children may observe their parents' injuries, distress, and depression or they might witness the police arresting the abusive person. Even when children are away from the family home and involved in activities at school or with friends, many of them describe a situation of being 'physically outside the home but emotionally and mentally inside it'.[1] Their ongoing preoccupation with the lack of safety in their home can result both in detachment from normal childhood activities and premature development of adult insights and responsibilities.[1,2]

Even when a parent separates from their abusive partner, children may still fear that the ex-partner will return to the family and recommence their abusive behaviour. Once a separation has occurred children may find that they move from the periphery of abusive incidents to the centre of parental disputes.[16] For those children who are able to end all contact with the abuser, many report that they still have to live with a 'history of abuse' as part of their life story.[1]

PREVALENCE OF CHILDREN'S INVOLVEMENT IN IPA

Although there are currently no reliable prevalence estimates, research findings to date indicate that children live in a large number of homes where IPA occurs. A national representative survey of the experience of IPA amongst a random sample of 6,300 Australian women found that 61% of the women who reported abuse by a current partner had children in their care and 38% of these women said that their children had witnessed the abuse.[17] An even greater number of women reported abuse in a previous relationship and 46% of this group indicated that their children had witnessed the abuse. Moreover, 50% of the women who reported that they had experienced abuse by a previous partner indicated that they ended the relationship because of this abuse or threats of abuse towards their children.

A study of five cities in the USA also confirmed that children were present in many households where IPA had occurred and that young children (0–5 years) were over-represented.[18] Findings indicated that young children were also more likely to be exposed to multiple incidents of IPA than older children. This same study examined whether IPA occurred in the context of arguments about children (e.g. disputes over lunch money for children, attention children received, or illness in children). Results indicated that children were identified as being a factor in the eruption of IPA in, on average, 19.8% of households. The two cities which tracked whether the call was made to the police by a child reported percentages of 11 and 12%, indicating that at least 1 in 10 calls to police were made by a child.

A study of former refuge residents in Australia found that despite their vulnerability, even the very young attempt to intervene in IPA.[9,19] Among the 54 children aged 3–6 years in the study, 39% displayed fear or *fright* responses culminating in emotional distress (e.g. crying, screaming) during an abusive incident. Sixteen (30%) children exhibited *fight* responses and intervened to protect their mother by either giving verbal instructions (e.g. 'stop hitting mummy') or physically hitting the abusive parent (e.g. a three-year-old boy stabbed his father in the leg with a bread-and-butter knife). Seven (13%) children adopted *flight* responses and withdrew to a different room. Some children attempted to distract their parents or acted protectively towards younger siblings.

THE IMPACT OF IPA ON CHILDREN

The last two decades have witnessed the rapid emergence of research on the effects of IPA on children's adjustment and several comprehensive reviews of the literature have been published.[3,20,21] The majority of studies are quantitative but a few qualitative studies have been published in recent years.[1] However, studies in this field have experienced many methodological limitations.[22]

Much of our current knowledge has been obtained from interviews with mothers and older children living in refuges. This is a problem for two reasons. Firstly, refuge children are not representative of all children who have experienced IPA. Secondly, research and clinical reports have indicated that mothers are not always aware of the extent of their children's exposure to IPA or the level of distress that children experience when these events occur.[2,23] The small sample sizes and retrospective nature of many studies have limited the interpretability of many findings.[22] Researchers have also failed to control for a range of additional risk factors (e.g. substance abuse, child abuse) which are often present in families where there is IPA. The focus has largely been on children with problems as opposed to a broader examination of children who exhibit resilience.[24,25] Ultimately, researchers still need to explore more refined questions such as 'Which children fare well, and which do not, and why?'

Behavioural and emotional problems

Results from published studies suggest that there is a fairly consistent relationship between IPA and externalizing behaviour problems in many of the children sampled from refuge or clinical populations. The percentages of children with behaviour problems have ranged from 25 to as high as 75% in these studies.[3,26] Typical externalizing behaviours have included aggressive behaviour, attention problems, delinquent and destructive behaviour, and hyperactivity. Similarly, research on children's emotional adjustment suggests that children living with IPA are at greater risk for the development of internalizing problems, although the results across studies are not always consistent for type of problem, gender, and age.[3] Percentages of refuge children with emotional problems have ranged from 35 to as high as 75%, and these problems have included anxiety, withdrawal, depression, psychosomatic complaints, separation anxiety, and sleep disturbances.[9,26,27]

Mental health, psychobiological, and neurodevelopmental problems

Exposure to IPA has also been linked to symptoms of psychological trauma. One study of 64 children aged between 7 and 12 years found that, although only 13% of the children qualified for a full post-traumatic stress disorder (PTSD) diagnosis, larger numbers suffered from traumatic symptoms such as intrusive and unwanted remembering of the traumatic events (52%); traumatic avoidance (19%); and traumatic arousal symptoms (42%).[28] Another prospective study which examined the use of mental health services by children (aged 4–8 years) found that having a mother who had been physically abused doubled the odds of mental health service use in the year after the baseline interview.[29]

More recently there have been concerns that children's responses to repetitive trauma from prolonged severe IPA may be accompanied by lasting changes in neurotransmitter functions in the brain. While this has not yet been examined in children, adults diagnosed with PTSD have an increased output of specific neurotransmitters that are believed to underlie symptoms such as attention and memory problems, mood fluctuations, and increased startle responses.[30] New knowledge about the vulnerability of the developing brain to prolonged traumatic stress also suggests that early experiences of trauma can interfere with the development of the subcortical and limbic areas of the brain, resulting in extreme anxiety, depression, and/or an inability to form healthy attachments to others.[31,32]

Physical health and development problems

A range of health problems have been reported among children living with IPA.[33] One study of preschool children living in a refuge reported that 35% had speech problems, 23% were enuretic, 11.5% had entered the refuge with allergies, and nearly 20% of the children had not been immunized for childhood diseases.[34] Another study reported that refuge children evidenced a number of medical problems, including prematurity and/or low birthweight, speech articulation and hearing difficulties, and a higher than average number of serious accidents. Similarly a survey of 148 children (0–15 years) living in refuges in Wales identified that one-fifth (19%) of the children less than five years old had delayed or questionable development on a developmental screening tool.[35] Almost one-third (30%) of the children for whom child health system data were available had incomplete immunization.

A review of the medical records of 139 children (aged two weeks to 17 years) who presented at a paediatric hospital with injuries resulting from IPA provided insights into the types and patterns of injuries that children can experience in this situation.[4] Although the mean age of the children was five years, 48% were younger than two years; 33% were younger than 12 months, and 10% were younger than one month. The most common mechanism of injury was a direct hit (36%) and 39% of the children were injured during attempts to intervene in IPA. The majority of the injuries were to the head (25%), face (19%), and eyes (18%) with younger children sustaining more head and facial injuries than older children. Medical intervention was indicated in 43% of the children, with 9% requiring hospital admission and 2% needing surgical or intensive care intervention.

Social competence

A small number of studies have investigated the effects of IPA on children's social competence.[36–38] One study investigated the social problem-solving abilities of children (aged 5–8 years) who witnessed IPA but were not themselves abused, compared with children from families where there was no IPA.[37] A measure was used to examine a range of social–cognitive skills and problem resolution strategies in peer and parental conflict situations. Results indicated that children from violent homes had greater difficulty identifying social problem situations and understanding the thoughts and feelings of those involved. Secondly, they tended to choose either passive (e.g. wishing for something to change, resolution by another's action) or aggressive (e.g. use of physical force) strategies to resolve interpersonal conflict and were less likely to choose assertive strategies (e.g. direct discussion, mutual compromise).

Another study that examined social competence utilized a stratified sample that included a refuge group, intact families where there was intimate partner violence, an intact group of families where there was verbal abuse but no physical violence, and a group of families where there was no verbal or physical abuse.[38] Surprisingly, children from families where there were higher levels of violence were rated as socially more competent by their mothers. Social sensitivity may have been advanced in these children due to their need to monitor adult behaviour to ensure their own protection from IPA.

LONGER-TERM EFFECTS OF IPA

Research which sheds some light on possible long-term effects includes retrospective studies involving adults who were exposed to IPA in childhood.[39] One study involving a non-clinical sample of college students found that young women who had witnessed IPA were significantly more depressed and aggressive than the women who had not.[40] Another study of 550 male and female college students found that, among women, childhood exposure to IPA was related to depression, trauma-related symptoms, and low self-esteem.[41] For men, exposure to IPA was associated with trauma-related symptoms. These relationships were statistically independent of reported parental alcohol abuse and divorce, but trauma-related symptoms depended, in part, on the co-occurrence of child abuse.

A retrospective survey of 1,452 undergraduate students found that 14% reported witnessing at least one incident of physical IPA during their childhood.[42] Both the young adult males and females who witnessed physical IPA reported higher levels of current psychological distress than a comparison group who had not witnessed physical IPA. This group difference remained after controlling for child abuse and parental divorce, socioeconomic status, alcoholism, and verbal discord. Additional analyses found that the effects of IPA were intensified when the aggression was serious enough to require external assistance for the victim and when the parent of the same sex was seen being victimized.

Research involving 8,629 participants examined the relationship of childhood physical abuse or sexual abuse, or growing up with an abused mother, to the risk of being a victim of IPA for women or a perpetrator for men.[43] Results indicated that each of the three violent childhood experiences increased the risk of victimization or perpetration of IPA approximately twofold. Among participants who had all three forms of violent childhood experiences, the risk of victimization and perpetration was increased 3.5-fold for women and 3.8-fold for men.

Research focused on juvenile and adult crime has also indicated that exposure to IPA is related to violent criminal behaviour in juveniles and adults, with this relationship being strongest for children who have witnessed extreme and/or routine violence.[44,45] While these studies suggest that some children who have been exposed to IPA will repeat this behaviour as adults, reviews of the research indicate that the majority do not.[46] The important issue appears to be that each child will have suffered, responded, or coped in a different way and some children appear to be more resilient than others.

FACTORS WHICH INFLUENCE CHILDREN'S COPING AND ADJUSTMENT

Research suggests that approximately 25–75% of children from refuge and clinical samples exhibit a clinical level of adjustment problems. It is likely that children's different reactions and their short-term and longer-term adjustment are related to a complex combination of child and family factors. This section briefly discusses a number of these key factors so that health practitioners will be aware of the issues that should be considered in any assessment of a child's unique responses to IPA.

Cumulative stresses: child abuse and parental alcohol abuse

Children living with IPA commonly experience a number of other stresses in their family.[9,13,47] For example, research suggests that child abuse is at least 15 times more likely to occur in families where IPA is present.[48] More severe levels of IPA appear to increase the probability of child abuse by the aggressive partner as well as the severity of the abuse that the children are likely to experience.[49] While research also suggests that abused women are more likely to be physically abusive towards their children, this relationship is stronger for the abusive partner than for abused women.[13] Research on children who have experienced both IPA and child abuse indicates that these children exhibit more emotional distress and behaviour problems than non-abused witnesses.[26,50] Similarly, substance abuse often coexists with IPA and can further exacerbate the negative impact of exposure to IPA.[27] Clinical literature highlights that children living with 'family secrets' like IPA or parental substance abuse are burdened with feelings of shame as well as the responsibility for helping their parents to deal with these problems.[2]

Parenting factors

The role that children play in the family and the quantity and quality of support children receive from parents are also factors that have the potential to positively or negatively influence children's ability to cope with IPA. While it is often assumed that mothers who have experienced IPA will exhibit diminished parenting capacity, a number of studies have found that children report that their mothers are a significant source of support.[51] Other studies have reported that IPA contributes to parental depression and stress which may adversely affect the level of support children receive.[52] For example, one study of adolescents in families where there was IPA reported less family emphasis on personal growth through social and recreational activities, less enjoyable time spent together, less family emphasis on personal independence, high parental control, and low organization in their family.[53]

One study which investigated the effects of IPA on women recruited through a refuge identified three main effects on parenting.[19] A quarter of the women reported that they were more verbally or physically aggressive towards their children prior to their separation from the abusive partner. A further 25% reported that their discipline and care of their children became inconsistent and erratic. Some women were virtually forced into neglecting their children by partners who demanded their exclusive attention. The other half of the women indicated that protection of their children was a key aspect of their parenting while living with their abusive partner. Some mothers reported that they tried to compensate for the abusive home environment by being lenient about the demands and pressures they placed on their children. Others indicated that their protectiveness consisted of vigilant monitoring of their children's behaviour in order to control or suppress behaviours which might provoke or irritate their partner. While such responses can be protective, prolonged lenient or controlling responses to children's behaviours and emotions can contribute negatively to the development of adjustment problems over time.

Developmental issues

How children react to and cope with IPA can be influenced by the developmental issues being addressed at the time they experience these traumatic events.[54,55] For example, a two-year-old male child who has witnessed the abuse of his mother could experience separation anxiety and become preoccupied by concerns about maternal abandonment and emotional unavailability. These anxieties may result in clinging behaviour, anxious attachment, language regression, and disruption in toilet training. A male child in middle childhood, on the other hand, may become attuned to the power that the abusive partner holds to induce submission to their demands. This may manifest itself in play behaviour and social interactions which attempt to grapple with the issue of mastery and control versus helplessness and inferiority.[56]

IPA can also generate conflicted loyalties in children where IPA involves their parents. For some children loving the abusive parent can feel like betraying the parent who is being victimized. Children's identification process can become conflicted and some children will be anxious about identifying with the parent who is being abused for fear that they too will be hit. Alternatively, some children may identify with the abusive parent to reduce the extent of their fears about personal safety.[57] Identification with the abusive parent's behaviour and attitudes can then result in children modelling and learning aggressive ways of interacting that may impede the development of empathy.[36]

Children's developmental stages will also influence their perspectives of stressful events such as IPA.[56] For example, children between the ages of 9 and 12 begin to view IPA in a more complex way than younger children. Children of this age group are likely to understand more about the intentions behind an abusive act. As a consequence of this increased understanding they can begin to feel more responsible for the abuse leading to worries such as 'Is it my fault?', 'How do I stop it?', 'When will it happen again?' An adolescent, on the other hand, has the capacity to take a third-person perspective and is more likely to recognize that there is little that they can do about IPA. While this means that some adolescents are less likely to blame themselves for IPA, feelings of hopelessness and powerlessness may develop and result in depression, suicidal thoughts, self-harming, and running away behaviours.[1]

Child characteristics: gender, age, and temperament

Gender should be considered a relevant factor but consideration needs to be given to the fact that there will be differences within, as well as between, the responses of girls and boys. While some studies have found that boys exhibited significantly more behavioural problems than girls and girls had significantly more emotional problems than boys, other studies have reported that both boys and girls have exhibited a concerning level of externalizing and internalizing behaviour problems.[3] With these qualifications in mind, it is important to acknowledge that in most cases what children are witnessing is male domination and female subordination, and many children's developing gender identities will be affected in some way.[58]

Age is another characteristic which has been studied in research on children exposed to IPA.[3] Studies report varied results, with some finding that younger children exhibit more behavioural and emotional problems and others finding that older children exhibit more adverse adjustment outcomes. Despite the lack of consistent evidence of age differences, practitioners report that tailoring therapeutic interventions to account for the developmental level of children is a more useful framework than differentiating interventions by children's gender.[11,56]

Temperament is another factor which can buffer children from adverse experiences or increase their risk of poor adjustment. Child development research suggests that children with 'easy' temperaments are sensitive to the positive aspects and less responsive to the more negative aspects of their social environment.[59] Indeed, a study involving refuge children aged 7–13 years found that children with an easy temperament had significantly lower levels of emotional and behavioural problems.[60]

Ethnicity

Few studies have addressed the role of ethnicity and culture. One study involving a large, racially and socioeconomically diverse sample group found that Asian-Americans reported significantly higher internalizing scores compared to Caucasians, whereas African-Americans reported significantly lower internalizing scores compared to Caucasians.[61] Another study conducted in the United Kingdom with a sample group of children from ethnically and culturally diverse backgrounds reported that children from minority cultural groups were better adjusted when they were able to remain in their community and obtain support from extended family.[62]

Dimensions of IPA and children's adjustment

IPA can vary in frequency, intensity or severity, duration, content, and resolution and can be overt or covert, chronic or sporadic, and some of these dimensions may be more specifically connected to child adjustment problems.[63] Studies which have considered the differential impact of specific aspects of IPA suggest that both the frequency and intensity are important.[64,65] Similarly, IPA which involves children is likely to be more distressing and thus may be more closely related to behaviour problems. The content of abusive incidents may also relate to children's emotional problems as it is linked to their attributions of blame and responsibility.[63] Moreover, the period of time over which children have been exposed to IPA is believed to influence their adjustment. For example, research findings have led to speculation that prolonged IPA results in parenting that is less sensitive, which in turn contributes to children's adjustment problems.[66]

Children's perceptions of IPA

There is also increasing evidence that children play an active role in the construction of their experiences and that children's interpretation of stressful events is critical for determining its impact upon them.[63] Researchers have begun to investigate whether the stress of IPA is mediated by children's appraisals of it, which are, in turn, shaped by characteristics of the abuse (e.g. intensity, frequency) and contextual factors (e.g. the emotional climate of the family). One study involving 60 children aged 8–12 years reported that those who perceived IPA to be more frequent and intense had significantly more emotional and behavioural problems according to their mothers' reports and their own reports. Children's attribution of perceived threat and self-blame was also higher when the IPA was more severe than when it was less intense. The children with higher scores for perceived threat and self-blame reported significantly more depression and significantly lower self-esteem scores.[67]

Although the significance of children's appraisals needs further investigation, there is increasing evidence that children's interpretation of IPA can influence the subsequent psychological and behavioural effects of these events. Some children may be able to emotionally distance themselves and be less likely to blame themselves. An important compensatory factor for children exposed to IPA may be their cognitive reorganization of experienced events, whether this occurs naturally or with therapeutic assistance.

IDENTIFICATION, ASSESSMENT, AND THERAPEUTIC INTERVENTION

An initial challenge to the provision of support and therapeutic services is the identification of children who are living with IPA. Once these children have been identified, their individual circumstances and needs can be assessed to determine whether intervention is necessary, and if so, which services are most appropriate. Key issues for health professionals involved in the identification, assessment, and treatment of children living with IPA are discussed in this section.

Identification

Rarely will physical injury or a direct disclosure of IPA by a child or a concerned parent be a presenting complaint. Rather, children living with IPA will present in any of a number of ways. Some children will present with many symptoms while others will have none (e.g. the 'supergood' child).

Indicators in infants and young children include:

- Growth and development problems (e.g. growth retardation, failure to thrive, developmental delay).
- Irritability, disruption to sleeping or eating behaviours.
- Disrupted attachment, separation anxiety.
- Evidence of fear or terror (e.g. screaming, stuttering, hiding).

Indicators in school age children include:

- Aggressive behaviour and language.
- Acting out or delinquent behaviours (e.g. cruelty to animals).
- Attention deficit hyperactivity disorder.
- Anxious, withdrawn, or hypervigilant behaviour.
- Depression, negative self-concept.
- Learning problems or disability.
- Bedwetting, psychosomatic problems.

Indicators in adolescents include:

- School failure or refusal.
- Running away, homelessness, delinquent or antisocial behaviours.
- Anxiety or depression, self-harming or suicidal behaviours.
- Being protective of parent and/or younger siblings.

Where these developmental, behavioural, or emotional problems are reported or observed in children, health practitioners should be alerted to the possibility that they may be the effects of IPA. In order to be able to ask a parent about the existence of IPA while undertaking a child health assessment, health practitioners will usually need to have established good rapport with the parent. Using a non-judgemental approach, health practitioners can indicate to a parent that IPA is an acceptable and normative topic of discussion when undertaking a child health assessment. This should only be done where appropriate and safe for the parent. When a disclosure is made the health practitioner should listen to and validate the disclosure and emphasize the unacceptability of IPA. The disclosure of IPA and any injuries on the child should be documented and the child's safety assessed.

Ideally, health care settings should ensure that they have developed and implemented guidelines for identifying and responding to disclosures of IPA. Even when these protocols are in place both mothers and children may be fearful that disclosure of IPA will result in repercussions that may further jeopardize the safety of family members. In these situations health professionals may need to build a trusting relationship over a period of time before children or their abused parent will make a disclosure and accept professional assistance. Once IPA has been identified, health professionals can play a significant role through the provision of support, appropriate referrals, and advocacy for children and their abused parent (see Chapter 9).

Assessment

A thorough assessment should explore the nature and duration of children's experiences of IPA and child abuse, their perceptions of, and involvement in, abusive incidents, and their current family circumstances, including the support and safety provided by the abused parent. Where children are interviewed, ideally this would be conducted by a child therapist using a focused clinical interview. A number of therapeutic interview strategies and protocols have been published that provide useful guides to this method.[2,68,69] If appropriate, this information can be supplemented by data about children's symptoms and experiences from other sources such as parents and teachers. Where children's health and development appear to have been affected by IPA, medical assessments by a paediatrician and child psychiatrist may be appropriate. Subsequent recommendations for intervention will be influenced by a thorough understanding of each child's unique circumstances and needs.

Therapeutic intervention

An initial goal of therapeutic intervention with children should be to promote frank discussion of their experiences as this provides a cathartic and healing experience, breaks the silence of family secrets, and begins to allow the child to integrate their experiences into their understanding of themselves and their world.[70] Therapeutic interventions should assist children to understand that while they cannot control IPA and should avoid becoming involved in IPA they do have control over their own thoughts and feelings about these events. Therapy can assist children to learn both control over their own behaviour and positive ways of coping with the difficulties they face, including symptoms which are affecting their physical and mental health.[70]

Effective intervention planning with children must be based upon an adequate assessment of safety and risk factors and should be consistent with the differential needs of children. Where children are still living in a dangerous environment, it is imperative that therapists work with the non-abusing parent to obtain safety for herself and her children. Without an adequate level of safety, children are not only placed at increased risk of victimization themselves but will also only obtain limited benefits from therapy.[71] Two further goals of therapy should be to reinforce the emotional bonds between children and their non-abusing parent and to make the parent aware of the connection between IPA and their children's behaviour, development, health, and well-being.[70] Recognizing the impact of IPA on children is often crucial to the victim's decision to leave the abusive situation.

Children's relationship with the perpetrator can also be a source of confusion, distress, and sadness, especially when this person is a parent figure. Therapeutic interventions should assist children to deal with these feelings, including any issues that might arise from conflicted loyalties.[72] Where health professionals identify that children have also experienced child abuse, they should adhere to any mandatory reporting laws or duty of care policies that govern their clinical practice and be prepared to work with child protection services if an investigation of suspected abuse proceeds.

To date, the focus of intervention with children has largely been on the development of group therapy programmes and, to a lesser extent, casework or psychotherapy approaches.[72–74] Unfortunately, controlled studies evaluating the effectiveness of these interventions are limited, but follow-up interviews with therapy participants and their mothers suggest that individual and group therapy interventions have positive effects. Groups have generally been a favoured method of intervention because they reduce children's isolation and can assist them to achieve important developmental tasks. They are, however, not appropriate for severely traumatized children, who have complex needs that would be better served by individual treatment.[1] For this particular group of children, many clinicians have adapted techniques used to treat PTSD in children while others have used psychodynamic approaches aimed at treating mother–child pairs.

SUMMARY

Large numbers of children live with IPA and these experiences can impact on their health and development. It is important that health practitioners increase their efforts to identify children who are living with IPA. Similarly, practitioners who identify abused women must make appropriate referrals so that children can be assessed and treated. Increased identification will require an expansion in services to this population of children and a need for greater coordination and communication between child health and adult health service systems. Clinicians and researchers also need to continue their efforts to develop and evaluate assessment techniques that promote the identification of children's individual needs. Finally, a greater focus on evaluation of treatment programmes will provide key information about effective treatment methods and the long-term effects of therapeutic intervention with children exposed to IPA.

REFERENCES

1. Blanchard A. Caring for child victims of domestic violence. Wangara, Western Australia: Nandina Press; 1999.
2. Jaffe P, Wolfe D, Wilson S. Children of battered women. Newbury Park, CA: Sage; 1990.
3. Kolbo JR, Blakely EH, Engleman D. Children who witness domestic violence: a review of empirical literature. J Interpers Violence 1996; 11(2):281–293.
4. Christian CW, Scribano DO, Seidl T, et al. Pediatric injury resulting from family violence. Pediatrics 1997; 99(2):1–4.
5. Webb E, Shankleman J, Evans MR, et al. The health of children in refuges for women victims of domestic violence: cross sectional descriptive survey. BMJ 2001; 323:210–213.
6. Campbell JC, ed. Empowering survivors of abuse: health care for battered women and their children. Thousand Oaks, CA: Sage; 1998.
7. Graham-Bermann SA, Edlesen JL, eds. Domestic violence in the lives of children: the future of research, intervention, and social policy. Washington, DC: American Psychological Association; 2001.
8. Groves B, Zuckerman B, Marans S, et al. Silent victims: children who witness violence. JAMA 1993; 269:262–264.
9. Smith JL, O'Connor I, Berthelsen D. The effects of witnessing domestic violence on young children's psycho-social adjustment. Aust Soc Wk 1996, 49(4):5–12.
10. Fantuzzo JW, Mohr WK, Prevalence and effects of child exposure to domestic violence. Future Child 1999; 9(3):21–30.
11. Morley R, Mullender A. Domestic violence and children: what do we know from research? In: Mullender A, Morley R, eds. Children living with domestic violence:

putting men's abuse of women on the child care agenda. London: Whiting & Birch; 1994:23–42.

12. Mullender A, Morley R, eds. Children living with domestic violence: putting men's abuse of women on the child care agenda. London: Whiting & Birch; 1994.

13. Edleson JL, Mbilinyi LF, Beeman SK, Hagemeister AK. How children are involved in adult domestic violence: results from a four-city telephone survey. J Interpers Violence 2003; 18(1):18–32.

14. Ross SM. Risk of physical abuse to children of spouse abusing parents. Child Abuse Negl 1996; 20(7):589–598.

15. Brandon M, Lewis A. Significant harm and children's experiences of domestic violence. Child Fam Soc Wk 1996; 1:33–42.

16. Hester M., Humphries J, Pearson C, et al. Domestic violence and child contact. In: Mullender A, Morley R, eds. Children living with domestic violence: putting men's abuse of women on the child care agenda. London: Whiting & Birch; 1994:102–121.

17. Women's safety Australia. Canberra: Australian Bureau of Statistics. Catalogue No. 4128.0; 1997.

18. Fantuzzo J, Boruch R, Beriama A, et al. Domestic violence and children: prevalence and risk in five major US cities. J Am Acad Child Adolesc Psychiatry 1997; 36(1):116–122.

19. Smith JL, Berthelsen D, O'Connor I. Child adjustment in high conflict families. Child Care Health Dev 1997; 23(2):113–133.

20. Osofsky JD. Children who witness domestic violence. Society for Research in Child Development: Social Policy Report 1995; 9(3):1–16.

21. Laing L. Children, young people and domestic violence. Australian Domestic & Family Violence Clearinghouse: Issues Paper 2000; 2:1–28.

22. Fantuzzo JW, Lindquist CU. The effects of observing conjugal violence on children: a review and analysis of research methodology. J Fam Violence 1989; 4(1):77–94.

23. O'Brien M, John RS, Margolin G, et al. Reliability and diagnostic efficacy of parents' reports regarding children's exposure to marital aggression. Violence Vict 1994; 9:45–62.

24. Hughes HM, Graham-Bermann SA, Gruber G. Resilience in children exposed to domestic violence. In: Graham-Bermann SA, Edlesen JL, eds. Domestic violence in the lives of children: the future of research, intervention, and social policy. Washington, DC: American Psychological Association; 2001:67–90.

25. Kolbo JR. Risk and resilience among children exposed to family violence. Violence Vict 1996; 11(2):113–128.

26. Sternberg KJ, Lamb ME, Greenberg C, et al. Effects of domestic violence on children's behaviour problems and depression. Dev Psychol 1993; 29(1):44–52.

27. Spaccarelli S, Sandler IN, Roosa M. History of spouse violence against mother: correlated risks and unique effects in child mental health. J Fam Violence 1994; 9(1):79–98.

28. Graham-Bermann SA, Levendosky AA. Traumatic stress symptoms in children of battered women. J Interpers Violence 2003; 13(1):111–128.

29. Plichta SB, McCue Horwitz S, Leventhal JM, et al. Use of mental health services by children of physically abused women. J Dev Behav Pediatr 1994; 15(3):186–197.

30. Rossman RB. Longer term effects of children's exposure to domestic violence. In: Graham-Bermann SA, Edlesen JL, eds. Domestic violence in the lives of children: the future of research, intervention, and social policy. Washington, DC: American Psychological Association; 2001:35–65.

31. Perry BD. Incubated in terror: neurodevelopmental factors in the 'cycle of violence.' In: Osofsky JD, ed. Children in a violent society. New York: Guildford Press; 1997:124–149.

32. Shore R. Rethinking the brain: new insights into early development. New York: Families and Work Institute; 1997.

33. Hughes HM. Research with children in shelters: implications for clinical services. Child Today 1986; 15:21–25.

34. Stagg V, Wills GD, Howell M. Psychopathology in early childhood witnesses of family violence. Top Early Child Spec 1989; 9(2):73–87.

35. Westra B, Martin HP. Children of battered women. Matern Child Nurs J 1981; 10:41–54.

36. Hinchley F, Gavelek J. Empathic responding in children of battered mothers. Child Abuse Negl, 1982; 6:395–401.

37. Rosenberg MS, Rossman BB. The child witness to marital violence. In: Ammerman RT, Hersen M, eds. Treatment of family violence: a sourcebook. New York: John Wiley; 1990:183–210.

38. Rossman BB, Rosenberg MS. Family stress and functioning in children: the moderating effects of children's beliefs about their control over parental conflict. J Child Psychol Psychiatry 1992; 33(4):699–715.

39. Cappell C, Heiner RB. The intergenerational transmission of family aggression. J Fam Violence 1990; 15(2):135–152.

40. Forsstrom-Cohen B, Rosenbaum A. The effect of parental marital violence on young adults: an exploratory investigation. J Marriage Fam 1985; (May):467–472.

41. Silvern L, Karyl J, Waelde L, et al. Retrospective reports of parental partner abuse: relationships to depression, trauma symptoms and self-esteem among college students. J Fam Violence 1995; 10(2):177–202.

42. Henning K, Leitenberg H, Coffey P, et al. Long-term psychological adjustment to witnessing interparental physical conflict during childhood. Child Abuse Negl 1997; 21(6):501–515.

43. Whitfield CL, Anda RF, Dube SR, et al. Violent childhood experiences and the risk of intimate partner violence in adults: assessment in a large health maintenance organization. J Interpers Viol 2003; 18(2):166–185.

44. Lewis DO, Pincus JH, Lovely R, et al. Biopsychosocial characteristics of matched sample of delinquents and nondelinquents. J Am Acad Child Adolesc Psychiatry 1987; 26:744–752.

45. Lewis DO, Shanock SS, Pincus JH, et al. Violent juvenile delinquents: psychiatric, neurological, psychological, and abuse factors. J Am Acad Child Adolesc Psychiatry 1979; 18:307–319.

46. Widom CS. Does violence beget violence? A critical examination to the literature. Psychol Bull 1989; 106(1):3–28.

47. Stanley J, Goddard C. The association between child abuse and other family violence. Australian Soc Wk 1993; 46(2):3–8.

48. Stacey W, Shupe A. The family secret. Boston: Beacon Press; 1983.

49. Bowker LH, Arbitell M, McFerron JR. On the relationship between wife beating and child abuse. In: Yllo K, Bograd M, eds. Feminist perspectives on wife abuse. Newbury Park, CA: Sage; 1988:158–174.

50. Hughes HM. Psychological and behavioural correlates of family violence in child witnesses and victims. Am J Orthopsychiatry 1988; 58(1):77–89.

51. Levendosky AA, Lynch SM, Graham-Bermann SA. Mothers' perceptions of the impact of woman abuse on their parenting. Violence Against Women 2000; 6(3):247–271.

52. Holden GW, Ritchie KL. Linking extreme marital discord, child rearing and child behaviour problems: evidence from battered women. Child Dev 1991; 62:311–327.

53. Resick PA, Reese D. Perception of family social climate and physical aggression in the home. J Fam Violence 1986; 1(1):71–83.

54. Roseby V, Johnston JR. In the name of the child: a developmental approach to understanding and helping children of conflicted and violent divorce. New York: Free Press; 1997.

55. Gaensbauer T. Developmental and therapeutic aspects of treating infants and toddlers who have witnessed violence. Zero to Three 1997:15–20.

56. Johnston JR, Roseby V. Clinical interventions with children of high conflict and violence: Part A. Theoretical framework, Paper presented at the 70th Annual Meeting of the American Orthopsychiatric Association, San Francisco; 1993:May 22.

57. Van Dalen A, Glasserman M. My father, Frankenstein: a child's view of battering parents. J Am Acad Child Adolesc Psychiatry 1997; 36(7):1005–1007.

58. Kelly L. The interconnectedness of domestic violence and child abuse: challenges for research, policy and practice. In: Mullender A, Morley R, eds. Children living with domestic violence: putting men's abuse of women on the child care agenda. London: Whiting & Birch; 1994:43–56.

59. Graham P, Rutter M, George S. Temperamental characteristics as predictors of behaviour disorders in children. Am J Orthopsychiatry 1973; 43:328–339.

60. O'Keefe M. Linking marital violence, mother-child/father-child aggression, and child behaviour problems. J Fam Violence 1994; 9(1):63–78.
61. O'Keefe M. The differential effects of family violence on adolescent adjustment. Child Adol Soc Wk J. 1996; 13:3–25.
62. Mullender A, Kelly L, Hague G, et al. Children's needs, coping strategies and understanding of woman abuse. Coventry: Economic and Social Research Council; 2000.
63. Grych JH, Fincham FD. Marital conflict and children's adjustment: a cognitive-contextual framework. Psychol Bull 1990; 108(2):26–290.
64. Hanson RF, Saunders BE, Kistner J. The relationship between dimensions of interparental conflict and adjustment in college-age offspring. J Interpers Violence 1992; 7(4):435–453.
65. Cummings EM, Vogel D, Cummings JS, et al. Children's responses to different forms of expression of anger between adults. Child Dev 1989; 60:1392–1404.
66. Jouriles EN, Pfiffner LJ, O'Leary SG. Marital conflict, parenting, and toddler conduct problems. J Abnorm Child Psychol 1988; 16:197–206.
67. Smith JL, Berthelsen D, O'Connor I. Children's appraisals of domestic violence: developmental implications. In: Berardo FM, Shehan CL, eds. Contemporary perspectives on family research, Vol. 1: Through the eyes of the child: revisioning children as active agents of family life. Stamford: JAI; 1999:247–272.
68. Arroyo W, Eth S. Assessment following violence-witnessing trauma. In: Peled E, Jaffe PG, Edleson JL, eds. Ending the cycle of violence: community responses to children of battered women. Thousand Oaks, CA: Sage; 1995:27–42.
69. Faller KC. Research and practice in child interviewing: implications for children exposed to domestic violence. J Interpers Violence 2003; 18(4):377–389.
70. Groves BA. Mental health services for children who witness domestic violence. Future Child 1999; 9(3):122–132.
71. Hurley DJ, Jaffe P. Children's observations of violence: II. Clinical implications for children's mental health professionals. Can J Psych 1990; 35(6):471–476.
72. Peled E. Intervention with children of battered women: a review of the current literature. Child Youth Services Review 1997; 19(4):277–299.
73. Peled E, Davis D. Groupwork with children of battered women: a practitioner's manual. Thousand Oaks, CA: Sage; 1995.
74. Roseby V, Johnston JR. High-conflict, violent, and separating families: a group treatment manual for school-age children. New York: Free Press; 1997.

Chapter 9

Managing the whole family when women are abused by intimate partners: challenges for health professionals

Angela Taft and Judy Shakespeare

It's hard to think of some of the men as abusers if you've been caring for them in other ways and really had no suspicion. I also think there's a tendency to minimise the violence and reassure yourself and the woman that, oh you know, its just bad temper.

I had one, just recently, how old was she? . . . Seven. And this mother was saying very clearly, it's not affecting the kid. And yet she was a bed wetter, and she had lots of the classic symptoms . . . She said, well, I hate it when mummy and daddy fight. And then I said what do you do? . . . I hide in the cupboard, and I take Jack with me. She had this whole behaviour, a way of protecting herself and her brother, who was about two, of getting into cupboards.

INTRODUCTION

Most guidelines, training, and information for health professionals about the identification and management of partner abuse have addressed only the female victims. This is appropriate and important, but overlooks the fact that men who abuse partners also attend health services and that the needs of children are often overlooked.[1] Chapters 7 and 8 explore the evidence of health damage to children who experience either direct abuse or who witness the abuse of their mother. This chapter discusses the prevalence within health services of men's reported abuse of partners, the characteristics of men who abuse, and gives guidance about men's identification, management, and referral. It also discusses the importance of enhancing parenting support to women and the management of the children and young people in these families. For health professionals who manage whole families, addressing intimate partner abuse (IPA) presents unique dilemmas.

Both victims and perpetrators suffer from complex comorbidities. There is considerable evidence that partner abuse is associated with significant mental disorders for victims[2] and their perpetrators.[3,4] Misuse of alcohol by the victims, survivors, and their perpetrators has been implicated in femicide.[5] Health care providers caring for women experiencing partner abuse, their partners, and their children need an index of suspicion about the possibility of partner abuse among those with mental disorder or substance abuse. They need skills for comprehensive assessment in these cases, an awareness of possible dilemmas, and the ability to collaborate with relevant services in the community. This chapter is especially relevant for health professionals in mental health, general/family practice, and drug and alcohol fields.

MEN WHO ABUSE THEIR PARTNERS

IPA is recognized worldwide and there is global consensus about the complex interrelated reasons for its existence.[6] Heise et al. proposed an ecological model, which outlined the reasons at the society, community, family, and individual levels. Both separately and together, these explain the abuse of female partners by men.[7] This conceptual model is clinically important because it (a) alerts clinicians that individual men's attitudes, cognition, and behaviour can be affected by societal and community norms, and (b) emphasizes that clinical interventions are important, but they are only one part of a wider system response in which legislation, policing, social sanctions, and community attitudes are critical to ending the violence.

Prevalence and comorbidities among men who abuse partners

There are methodological difficulties in interpreting men's self-reports of IPA in the community.[8-10] The most consistent evidence comes from studies of women's self-reported prevalence of lifetime exposure to victimization from male partners. These show prevalence rates of 10–69% globally, but in most developed countries the rate is about 20–25%.[6]

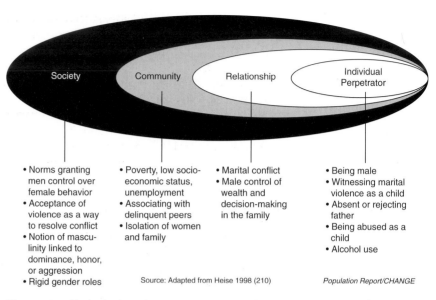

Society	Community	Relationship	Individual Perpetrator
• Norms granting men control over female behavior • Acceptance of violence as a way to resolve conflict • Notion of masculinity linked to dominance, honor, or aggression • Rigid gender roles	• Poverty, low socio-economic status, unemployment • Associating with delinquent peers • Isolation of women and family	• Marital conflict • Male control of wealth and decision-making in the family	• Being male • Witnessing marital violence as a child • Absent or rejecting father • Being abused as a child • Alcohol use

Source: Adapted from Heise 1998 (210)   Population Report/CHANGE

Figure 9.1   Ecological model of factors associated with partner abuse. (Reproduced from Heise, Ellsberg, Gottemoeller (1999), adapted from Heise (1998)[7] and reprinted with permission from Sage Publications (applied).)

Epidemiological evidence exists about high rates of violence among specific male populations, such as men in the Armed Forces, including veterans.[11] A recent study suggested that IPA is more prevalent among gay male than female couples.[12] More research is required, but health care providers should be aware of the potential for partner violence in this population.[13]

Limited evidence can be presented about the prevalence of partner abuse by male clients/consumers of health care services. In a small US study in family practice, 13.5% of male primary care patients reported abusing their partners, with 4.2% reporting severe abuse.[14] Oriel et al. suggest that male patients who were depressed, alcohol abusers, or childhood victims of abuse are more likely to abuse their partners. In an ethnographic study, Taft et al. found that male perpetrators presented to general practitioners (GPs) with depression, pain, substance abuse, and mental illness. In addition the men also attended for non-medical reasons, such as 'anger management' or 'wife-mandated' behaviour change.[1] Another small study found high levels of stress and self-inflicted injuries among batterers.[15] A study from Pittsburgh showed that of 133 abusive men in a behaviour change program, 42% had visited health care services in the preceding six months, and of these, the largest group (41%) had attended an emergency department.[16]

Several studies of male clients in drug and alcohol services have found an association between substance abuse and men's reported violence against their partners.[17,18] In addition, in one study of male perpetrators, the dangerousness and frequency of abusive behaviours increased as the severity of the substance abuse increased.[19] This does not mean that substance abuse causes partner abuse, but it is a significant risk factor.

In one study of homicide/suicide of 119 women victims, recent separation from an abusive partner was found to be the most prevalent precursor (41%), followed by a history of domestic violence (29%).[20] In this study 43% of children of the victim and/or perpetrator witnessed the homicide/suicide, or were in the immediate vicinity, or found a parent's body, or were killed themselves. Sharps and colleagues found an association between prior domestic abuse and use of health care services among victims and perpetrators of femicide. They argued that contacts with agencies, such as substance abuse and drug treatment programmes, offer potential opportunities for health care providers to prevent femicide.[21]

Profiles and heterogeneity among men who abuse

Profiling the characteristics of abusive men is a new field of research. There is disagreement about which factors are the most important clinically for predicting beneficial results from intervention.[22,23] It is clinically important to understand that men who abuse are heterogeneous. In the most comprehensive review of psychological studies of violent men, Holtzworth-Munroe et al. argue that different men require different forms of treatment.[24] They examined three dimensions of the violence:

- The severity and frequency of violence, including psychological and sexual abuse.
- The domain of violence – family-only, extra-familial, and/or criminal.
- The abusers' psychopathology or personality disorder.

They identified three types of perpetrator:

1. *The family-only group*, who engage in the least severe violence, the least violence outside the family, and least criminal behaviour.
2. *The borderline-dysphoric group*, whose violence is moderate to severe, who are violent outside the family, psychologically distressed with some borderline personality characteristics, and have problems with substance abuse.
3. *The generally violent-antisocial group*, who are moderately to severely violent against partners and with the most extra-familial violence and most criminal behaviour. This group were more likely to have an antisocial personality and substance abuse problems.

These broad three types and some subtypes have been found in other studies.[22,25] Mintz and Cornett agreed that it is clinically important to distinguish between male patients who abuse, as they might require different forms of management.[4] They argued that men might fall into one of three types:

- *'Cyclically emotional volatile perpetrators'*. Such men are emotionally dependent on their partner's presence. They have developed a pattern of escalating tension leading to aggression towards the partner, followed by a period of contrition, like the 'cycle of violence' first described by Lenore Walker and found among 60% of her respondents.[26-28]

- *'Over-controlling perpetrators'*. These men develop a pattern of control that relies more on psychological or emotional rather than physical abuse. Such men can be very compliant patients, often attend with their partners, and are unwilling to leave them alone.
- *'Psychopathic perpetrators'*. These men lack emotional engagement or feelings of remorse and are more likely to be involved in general violence and other criminal behaviour. Health care providers should not engage with these men in any attempt to manage their violence, for fear of their personal safety.

One of the most useful insights into clinically important characteristics of abusive men comes from a rigorous American study. In the largest American evaluation of mainly court-mandated perpetrator programmes, Gondolf tested 842 men for psychopathology, personality tendencies, and disorders.[29] He found a gradient ranging from low (56%), through moderate (29%), to severe (15%) levels of personality pathology, with a minority of men who needed referral for additional psychiatric help or close monitoring of violation of limits. However, he found less pathology than other studies had done and a notable trend towards narcissistic or antisocial personality among the majority of participants. Gondolf concluded that perpetrators act with a sense of entitlement, dominance, and self-centredness.

The study found no support for the proposition that perpetrators are characterized by borderline personality tendencies. Gondolf stated that *'these findings raise caution to characterizations that overly pathologize batterers and battering'*.[29] At the same time he suggested that *'the prevailing gender-based, cognitive-behavioural group treatment may, however, be appropriate for most men referred to batterer (men's behaviour change) programmes. It appears that although one size does not fit all, one size appears to fit most.'* The author emphasized that these programmes were located within the criminal justice system and were only one part of a system-wide response.[29] Clinicians should be aware that many men who abuse in the wider community may not be known to the criminal justice system, but they may nevertheless seek help for their health problems,[1,14] in which case clinicians may need to encourage women to seek legal and judicial protection.

Principles and goals of management

The major principles for health care providers when they manage abusive men should be the safety and well-being of women and children. The major management objectives are: to identify male patients/clients who abuse; to condemn the behaviour but not the man; to take a history, including his level of suicidality and weapon ownership, substance misuse, and mental health problems; to assist him to take responsibility for his behaviour and encourage him to make beneficial change. This could include referring him to a specialist men's behaviour change group and treating any comorbid problems. Whether or not the man is attending a court-mandated or voluntary behaviour change programme, clinicians can encourage and support his efforts to change, while at the same time monitoring the safety and welfare of victims and children.

Attitudinal barriers in health care professionals

Health care providers should be aware of common myths about men who abuse:

- *Perpetrators of partner abuse are all mentally ill.* While many perpetrators are depressed, even suicidal, and many have substance misuse problems, relatively few have serious mental illness.
- *Perpetrators cannot control their anger.* Many perpetrators are able to control their anger at work, and are only abusive in the home. These men are indistinguishable from other 'normal' members of society and could be playing prominent and respected roles in society.
- *Perpetrators are violent only when they are drunk.* While some men use alcohol to excuse their behaviour, many men with alcohol problems do not abuse their partners and others abuse partners when sober. The abuse of power and control is the problem, not the alcohol.

Taft et al. found that family doctors in their sample could hold a range of unhelpful attitudes towards their abusive male patients.[1] The GPs attitudes could be uncomprehending, hostile, and distancing, or doctors explained the behaviour as part of men's class, ethnicity, or genetic predisposition. Other doctors had difficulty accepting that a charming male patient they had known for years was abusing his partner. Both hostile and ambivalent responses to abusive male patients made it difficult for doctors to respond appropriately to the men's violence. When doctors distance themselves from abusive male patients, they can place greater responsibility on women to change their situation, irrespective of the women's ability to do so. Health care providers should reflect on their own attitudes to abusive male patients, but neither stereotype men from abusive backgrounds, nor avoid encouragement to change. Romans and colleagues state, 'It is important to remember most men experiencing negative pressures (such as abuse as a child, unemployment or mental health disorders) will not be physically aggressive. The intergenerational and social transmission of violence, although influential, can be avoided.'[30] They advise that there are several steps in effective intervention with which health professionals should be involved:

- recognize partner violence and identify the perpetrator;
- understand (but do not excuse) the perpetrator's actions;
- provide effective management of both victim and perpetrator.

Disclosure and confidentiality

If male patients present with, for example, alcohol problems, anger problems, injuries, or depression, health professionals can gently ask about how things are at home, or with their partner and family. They should suspect that if a man is abusive towards himself, with problem drinking, drug abuse, or self-harm, then abuse of others is also a possibility. In this situation funnelling questions may be useful,[31] progressing from broad ones about 'how are things at home' to more specific questions about specific acts and their consequences. For example 'What do you do when you're angry?', or 'You say you hit the wall when you're angry, how do your wife and children respond?' Alternatively, 'You say you just pushed her when you're angry, is that against a wall or downstairs? What impact did that have on her?' Men will often minimize their violence, especially to a professional. If you also see the victim, always ask her about the level of violence she has experienced and how she assesses its severity, frequency, and impact on herself and the children, so that you can gain her perspective.

If a woman has disclosed her partner's violence to a health service provider, this should not be raised with the man without her permission. There have been documented instances of well-meaning health practitioners doing this from genuine concern for the victim, but without her knowledge,[1,32] and it can result in physical punishment for her disclosure.

Managing men who abuse

The major goals in the management of men who abuse are monitoring everyone's safety and assisting the man to take responsibility for his violent or abusive behaviour, while expressing support for his efforts to change. Some men can be encouraged to seek change, while others cannot. Posters and leaflets offering advice or support to victims and perpetrators in the waiting room provide recognition of the issue and encouragement to talk about it. If a man discloses any form of violent behaviour, it is important to take a thorough history. Always check if his behaviours include harassment (constant calls to work to check up on her), stalking, social isolation, forced sex, threats or use of weapons, violence towards other family members or pets. Often men will excuse their behaviours by blaming others, mental illness, or alcohol intoxication.

Men who are depressed or suicidal should be managed appropriately. Separation, coupled with suicidal ideation, is dangerous for the whole family and needs careful monitoring. A man needs to understand the professional limits to confidentiality and if he has threatened his family or others to you, you may be required to report this to authorities in some countries, under a duty to protect (The Tarasoff warning).[33]

Men's behaviour change programmes

Male behaviour change groups were first encouraged by women's refuge workers responding to women who did not want to leave male partners, but wanted the violence to stop. These programmes are now funded in many developed countries as part of an overall response to domestic violence, although conditions under which they are provided differ. Most commonly, especially in the USA and UK, programmes are court-mandated. In some parts of the US, UK, and Australia, there are also voluntary programmes to which men can self-refer or be referred. In Australia, there is a national telephone counselling and referral service for men. These programmes are controversial because (a) their effectiveness is difficult to demonstrate, (b) there are limited funds and helping female victims may be perceived to be a more deserving cause, (c) the programmes use different theoretical models, and (d) there is a risk that women will falsely hope that their men will change, potentially compromising their safety.[22]

It is not easy to measure the effectiveness of such programmes. Many have a significant dropout rate. They are effective to a degree in reducing the violence for those who are retained in treatment, but they can be completely ineffective with up to a quarter of all men. Most groups combine cognitive–behavioural therapy and gender resocialization to change attitudes. Depending on the strength of legislation and effective policing in each context, the length and treatment style of groups seem to be equally effective. In comprehensive American and UK evaluations, the majority of women said their lives had been improved. The conclusions of the most rigorous evaluations recognize that such programmes have an important, but limited part to play in eliminating male partner violence against women.[29,34]

Not all men are ready for referral to a behaviour change programme, especially if they are not under a court order to attend. If they have accepted responsibility for their behaviours, clinicians can suggest a number of ways in which they can improve family relationships themselves, by reducing controlling or coercive behaviours. Options and encouragement to improve behaviours should be made at every opportunity. Health professionals are in a strong position of authority and influence if they express disapproval and zero tolerance of violent or abusive behaviour.

If a man has accepted responsibility for his behaviour, the next goal is referral to specialist behaviour change services or monitoring and supporting his involvement in any court-mandated groups. It is vital that health care providers are familiar with men's telephone support services if available, and contact details and accreditation of any voluntary men's behaviour change groups in the area. Such programmes should always include performance standards, support for victims, and evaluation, including victims' assessment of progress. If you refer a man to a behaviour change programme, it is important to monitor the reduction or increase in violence with his partner, who may base her decision to stay with him on his attendance at the group and risk further, possibly escalating abuse. One of the best catalysts for change is to ask abusive men whether they wish their children to grow up like them; they frequently do not. Discussing the impact of violence on children can be an important motivator to change.[35]

PARTNER VIOLENCE, PARENTING, CHILDREN, AND YOUNG PEOPLE

Chapter 7 outlines that the violence can commence or continue when the woman is pregnant, as an assault on the fetus, and continue through child infancy, early childhood, and adolescence. Chapter 8 describes the close relationship between IPA and child abuse and neglect, and outlines how witnessing or living in a house where there is violence between adults is associated with damage to children's physical and mental health, and social and educational well-being.

The cumulative impact of abuse can increase the health damage to children and young people, but such damage is not inevitable. Many children survive without harm because of a secure attachment to a non-violent parent or other significant carer.[36] Having someone to turn to for emotional support is important; this could be a friend, a grandparent, or other relatives.[37] Clinicians, especially family doctors, school nurses, or counsellors, who have an ongoing relationship with the child or young person, can play additional supportive roles, by coordinating support with a non-abusive parent and monitoring any changes in the frequency and severity of the current level of violence.

IPA and parenting

In addition to the social deprivation and isolation for the mother caused by IPA (whether or not she remains in the abusive relationship), she may suffer specific health problems related to the violence, which can impact on her ability to parent effectively in several ways:

- She is rendered less effective through tranquillizing medication.
- She is constantly 'walking on egg shells' to avoid violence.
- She is depressed.
- She is unable to keep herself or her children safe.
- She may be more likely to abuse the children herself.
- The children are more difficult to manage and older children may be abusing her.

The risks of depression among abused women are significantly increased. Golding found depression increased 3-fold, drug abuse 9-fold, alcohol abuse 15-fold, and suicide attempts 5-fold.[38,39] An abused woman may become passive and paralysed by her situation, which can also affect her ability to protect and parent her children, the so-called 'battered wife syndrome'.[27] Dubowitz discovered that there was a timing of effects among 419 mothers of children aged 6–7 years.[40] Mothers victimized during childhood and adulthood had poorer outcomes (maternal depression, harsher parenting, and more externalizing and internalizing behaviour problems in children) than mothers victimized in one period only, and more than women not victimized at all.

Managing when children are directly abused by the male partner

Studies of young people and children have identified the strategies mothers use to protect and support their children.[41] Men who abuse their partners often abuse their children as well. In many countries, clinicians are obliged to report suspected child abuse. Women, especially those with mental health disorders or involved in substance abuse, may be fearful that their children might be removed or that the father may gain their custody, by using their medical conditions in court against them. Often services will focus on a woman's inability to protect her children rather than condemning the man's violence, and thus fail to offer effective support. Edleson has argued that this continued focus on the mother is unfair.[41] He urges action to hold the perpetrator of violence accountable, rather than focusing on the mother's failure to protect her children. Too often, he argues, women are held accountable for society's failure to deal with violent men. Clinicians also need to be culturally sensitive and aware of the socio-cultural context and implications of decisions about child abuse and parenting. They can inquire, in a reassuring, non-judgemental, and supportive manner, about how victimized women are coping with parenting, and offer additional support.

If the health professional has made a thorough risk assessment, with the woman's full cooperation, supporting her is likely to be the most effective way of promoting the child's welfare.[42] Encouraging and supporting a woman to engage with the criminal justice system or other appropriate systems to help keep herself and her children safe is more constructive than blaming her for the lack of safety. This could be by helping her make safe choices for herself and her children or by providing practical information and sign-posting into multi-agency resources, such as refuges, or referral to social or legal services or the police.

A health professional should try to establish a trusting, open relationship in which a woman understands that you are trying to support her and her children in making safe choices, but be explicit about the obligations and limits to confidentiality under which health care professionals operate. Such cases are always time consuming, complex, different, and emotionally demanding for health care professionals. Sharing concerns and clarifying responsibilities with other involved colleagues within the primary care team, preferably with the non-abusive parent's consent, is to be encouraged.

Under the circumstances when a breach of confidentiality would be acceptable (because a child is at real risk), recognize that this could increase the danger to the woman, her child, and you or your colleagues, from the perpetrator. Try to engage the non-abusive partner in that discussion and support her, as this may be the 'final straw' that enables her to make the decision to leave. Whatever decision the woman makes, a health care worker must be confident that his or her action (e.g. referral to social services) will not place someone at greater risk of violence, especially the woman.

Talking to children who are living with IPA

Men who abuse their partners may not necessarily abuse their children directly, but witnessing violence is still a damaging experience for children. It is possible that neither parent may be aware of the detrimental impact the abuse is inevitably having on the children or young people. Asking about the impact of abuse on children is often a catalyst for either parent to make beneficial change. It is useful to try to make an opportunity to speak to the children themselves in confidence. Children often know much more then their parents think. Find out from them directly about their needs. It may not be helpful for them to stay in the family home. Offer them support and invite them to discuss the situation and their safety with you at any time. You could encourage them to tell other people that they trust, such as friends or grandparents, about what is happening in the home; discuss safety planning with them, where would they flee if they felt unsafe; and refer them to helpful services. If neither the mother nor the father has disclosed to you what is happening in the home, do not breach confidentiality, unless you have discussed this with the child first.

The impact of violence on young people

Research has demonstrated the impact of living with violence in the family on adolescent and teenage children. Such young people may leave home to escape the violence, may be depressed or suicidal, and may have difficulties with education and misuse drugs and alcohol.[41] Some young people may attempt to protect the victim and find themselves attacked as a result. Teenage children may assault a non-abusive parent: so-called child-parental violence (CPV).[43] In a US study, interviews with parents of American children aged 3–17 (parents 18–69) found that adolescent violence was worse against mothers than fathers, and was perpetrated especially by boys, who may identify with the abusive and more powerful father. The younger the child, the more CPV was associated with violence by parents. In the absence of parent-to-child violence, CPV was rare. If health care providers are aware that there is partner abuse in the home, they should ask about whether the young people feel safe, if their parents are safe, and about their mental and physical health and well-being. If a woman has disclosed partner abuse, she should be asked whether she is also experiencing violence from any of her children. She may need additional support from behaviour change services for adolescents.

Safety planning

Safety planning refers to a discussion with the non-abusive parent and/or the young people and children in the family about the following:

- Safe storage of contact details for helpful or emergency services, including police.
- Spare, hidden copies of the house or car keys.
- Copies of important documents such as passports, and marriage, immigration, and birth certificates.
- Secret storage of money for emergencies.
- Signals for the neighbours to call the police when necessary; for example, pulling down the blind halfway.

It is vitally important to discuss if the level of danger is serious or escalating. Campbell has written a guide to the difficult task of risk assessment for homicide.[44]

MANAGING ALL FAMILY MEMBERS

The major principles of health care provider management of all family members are the same: safety and confidentiality (unless there is the threat of homicide, suicide, or infanticide).

Balancing competing needs

All the family members, including the perpetrator and victims (including the children), could present to the same group of health care providers, although they may be seeing different colleagues. This requires providers to ensure that there is effective case management within their service. This may mean:

- Having a system for flagging increased danger, for example, a coloured flag in the files.
- Ensuring everybody inquires about the safety of the children.
- Family case management meetings.
- Effective protocols between the provider and other relevant services, for example, mental health, police, and legal services.
- Ensuring personal safety.

Managing the couple

Within primary care, providers may be in the difficult situation of caring for both the perpetrator and the abused. A consensus document from Canada felt that this was not necessarily a conflict of interest for doctors, but that they should feel free to refer to another physician if this was preferred.[45] It can be very difficult if a doctor has a long-standing professional or social relationship with a couple and the wife then discloses abuse. Health care providers may feel unable to provide support to both sides equitably, but each situation should be considered independently. The provider needs to make an explicit decision about whether s/he can or cannot continue to care for both parties and if s/he cannot, convey this clearly to both the perpetrator and the abused in a way that does not increase the danger to anyone, including her- or himself. However, a provider is ethically obliged to ensure that the perpetrator receives ongoing care and should facilitate referral to someone else. Collaborative case management between providers seeing partners and/or children, highlighting the principle of safety of victims, is encouraged.

Health care providers need to consider their own personal attitudes to either the victim or abuser that could be unhelpful: they may experience difficulty reframing the man as an 'abuser'; they may perceive that the victim has deserved the treatment, especially if she 'nags' or her behaviour is difficult. Victimization in childhood can leave a woman's personality damaged. Nevertheless all violence and abuse should be considered unacceptable and a professional empathy and good management offered to her. It is vital that health professionals maintain strict confidentiality when they are seeing both parties in a couple, so as not to endanger a woman further.

Couple or marital counselling is contraindicated

Health care providers are not usually trained to counsel couples when partner abuse is present in a relationship, and unless they are, they should avoid it.[46–48] Couple or marital counselling without such training can leave the victim vulnerable to further abuse. A woman is certainly powerless to make honest statements about the abuse in front of her abuser.

Enhancing the engagement of health professionals in multi–agency processes

Families living with partner abuse are complex, with comorbidities and involvement with many other community-based services, such as primary mental health care services, drug and alcohol services, child protection services, and probation or criminal justice services. This requires health professionals to collaborate in inter-sectoral and multi-agency processes, because their involvement can ensure integrated case management. This may be difficult for some health care providers; they may have anxieties about confidentiality; they may not have been trained or paid to engage in such processes. Some helpful models have been outlined.[49,50]

Recognizing your responsibility to contribute to inter-agency processes

British studies have demonstrated that clinicians currently attend very few child protection conferences and other professionals perceive this low level of involvement as a lack of commitment to inter-agency working.[51,52] Gondolf has outlined how differing theoretical models and treatment responses between mental health and domestic violence services can also contribute to misunderstanding in inter-agency processes.[49] However, clinicians have a responsibility in the joint decision-making about children. They can validate the health damage to adult and child victims and they have useful information to contribute for the benefit of the child. Time constraints make it difficult to attend conferences themselves, but they can contribute to the inter-agency process in several ways: they can ensure that the appropriate documentation is completed and available; they can brief others from the practice, such as nurses, to officially represent their views at the conference; if they know that the mother is experiencing IPA they can warn the conference that the parents should be seen separately, so that an objective and proper assessment can be made.

Resources

It is important that health care providers know about the support that other community-based services can provide and that they equip clients/patients with realistic expectations of what to expect. Patients are often fearful of what will happen if they accept a referral. They need to know about current waiting times. Often community-based services are under-resourced and overstretched. It may help to offer to make an assisted referral yourself, rather than expecting patients to approach a behaviour change or domestic violence service themselves.

Record-keeping and documentation

IPA and child protection issues should be documented in detail if a disclosure is made. In the UK it is recommended that only one set of records is kept within a practice team, so that all members of the team have access to identical information.[53] There is always a risk of inadvertent disclosure to the perpetrator if IPA and children's issues have been discussed, particularly with desktop computers in primary care. This could increase the danger to the woman and children. Practices need to decide how they will address the potential conflict between keeping details confidential from the perpetrator and protecting the children's interests by the accessibility of key information, for example to a locum who may not know the family.

The written records could be coded with a coloured sticker (with no wording) to indicate that additional sensitive information is held elsewhere and that any consulting doctor should seek it out. In a paperless practice there could be a coded entry on the 'current problems' screen. Of course, the practice would need to communicate the existence of such a tagging system to all locums or new members of the team via their practice induction folder, or the system will not work. Any letters to outside agencies, such as lawyers, should be written in the knowledge that they are likely to be made available to both sides in a case.

Training

Health professionals need training to increase their awareness, knowledge, understanding of family violence and attitudes about IPA and children's issues, and to identify and manage the 'Pandora's box' of intimate partner violence,[54] but they are traditionally reluctant to seek it. Although training programmes for IPA have not yet been adequately evaluated,[55] clinicians are encouraged to explore what is currently available and seek training to manage all members of family and to effectively coordinate their care.[1] (See Chapter 4 for a full discussion of training.)

The needs of high-risk and less accessible groups

Women and children living in refuges are the most easily identified high-risk group, who may have experienced both IPA and child abuse. Primary care professionals need to recognize that these individuals have a significant risk of mental health problems and they often have unmet health needs, such as immunizations or dental problems. They are a peripatetic population, whose accessibility to services may be transient, and they deserve proactive support and care from the practice.[56] Clinicians need to ensure the provision of primary care to refuges. Additional resources, such as counselling, need to be funded adequately.

There are particular language and cultural issues for ethnic minorities, especially in the situation when children are asked to act as interpreters. Practices need to be able to work with impartial interpreters routinely so that they are able to consult with women in confidence (see Chapter 11).

Children and mothers with disabilities may have particular difficulties when there is family violence; they may be dependent on the perpetrator for practical care or have established care packages at home that make it difficult to leave.

Safety in the practice

Lastly, clinicians need to examine their own safety employment law to ensure the safety of themselves and their staff. There is a need for open discussion about safety and confidentiality in the practice, and this may include the need for doubling up on some visits, especially if the perpetrator may be present.

SUMMARY AND CONCLUSION

This chapter has outlined the presenting symptoms, identification strategies, and management of male patients or clients who use violence against their partner; the impact this has on women's ability to parent effectively; and the protection of children and young people in the family. It has emphasized the important management principles of safety and confidentiality of women and children and the need for careful case management and inter-sectoral collaboration. It also encouraged clinicians to seek further training in order that they have the knowledge and skills for this critical task when it is necessary.

REFERENCES

1. Taft A, Broom DH, Legge D. General practitioner management of intimate partner abuse and the whole family: a qualitative study. BMJ 2004; 328:618–621.
2. Astbury J, Cabral M. Women's mental health: an evidence based review. Geneva: WHO; 2000.
3. Danielson KK, Moffitt TE, Caspi A, et al. Comorbidity between abuse of an adult and DSM 111-R mental disorders: evidence from an epidemiological study. Am J Psychiatry 1998; 155(1):131–3.
4. Mintz HA, Cornett FW. When your patient is a batterer: what you need to know before treating perpetrators of domestic violence. Postgrad Med 1997; 101(4):219–228.
5. Sharps PW, Campbell JC, Campbell D, et al. The role of alcohol use in intimate partner femicide. Am J Addiction 2001; 10(2):122–35.
6. Krug EG, Dahlberg LL, Mercy JA, eds. World report on violence and health. Geneva: WHO; 2002.
7. Heise LL. Violence against women: an integrated, ecological framework. Violence Against Women 1998; 4(3):262–290.
8. Ferrante A, Morgan F, Indermaur D, et al. Measuring the extent of domestic violence. Sydney: Hawkins Press; 1996.
9. Taft A, Hegarty KL, Flood M. Are men and women equally violent to intimate part-ners. Aust N Z J Public Health 2001; 25(6):498–500.
10. Straus M. Trends in cultural norms and rates of partner violence: an update to 1992. In: Stith SM, Straus MA, eds. Understanding partner violence: prevalence, causes, solutions. Minneapolis, MA: National Council on Family Relations; 1995:30–33.
11. Brewster AL, Milner JS, Mollerstrom WW, et al. Evaluation of spouse abuse treatment: description and evaluation of the Air Force Family Advocacy Programs for spouse physical abuse. Mil Med 2002; 167(6):464–9.
12. Tjaden P, Thoennes N, Allison CJ. Comparing violence over the lifespan in samples of same-sex and opposite-sex cohabitants. Violence Vict 1999; 14(4):413–25.
13. Burke LK, Follingstad DR. Violence and lesbian and gay relationships: theory, preva-lence, and correlational factors. Clin Psychol Rev 1999; 19(5):487–512.
14. Oriel KA, Fleming MF. Screening men for partner violence in a primary care setting: a new strategy for detecting domestic violence. J Fam Practice 1998; 46(6):493–8.
15. Gerlock AA. Health impact of domestic violence. Issues Ment Health Nurs 1999; 20(4):373–85.
16. Coben JH, Friedman DI. Healthcare use by perpetrators of domestic violence. J Emerg Med 2002; 22(3):313–317.
17. Easton CJ, Swan S, Sinha R. Prevalence of family violence in clients entering substance abuse treatment. J Subst Abuse Treat 2000; 18(1):23–8.
18. Chase KA, Farrell TJ, Murphy CM, et al. Factors associated with partner violence among female alcoholic patients and their male partners. J Stud Alcohol 2003; 64:137–149.
19. Brown TG, Werk A, Caplan T, et al. Violent substance abusers in domestic violence treatment. Violence Vict 1999; 14(2):179–90.

20. Morton E, Runyon CW, Moracco KE, et al. Partner homicide – suicide involving female homicide victims: a population based study in North Carolina, 1988 to 1992. Violence Vict 1998; 13(2):91–106.

21. Sharps PW, Koziol-McLean J, Campbell J, et al. Health care providers missed opportunities for preventing femicide. Prev Med 2001; 33(5):373–380.

22. Laing L. Responding to men who perpetrate domestic violence: controversies, interventions and challenges. Issues paper 7. Sydney: Australian Domestic and Family Violence Clearinghouse, University of New South Wales; 2002.

23. Eiskovits ZC, Edleson JL, Guttmann E, et al. Cognitive styles and socialised attitudes of men who batter: where should we intervene? In: Stith S, Straus M, eds. Understanding partner violence: prevalence, causes, consequences and solutions. Minneapolis, MA: National Council on Family Violence; 1995.

24. Holtzworth-Munroe A, Stuart GL. Typologies of male batterers: three subtypes and the differences among them. Psychol Bull 1994; 116(3):476–497.

25. Hamberger LK, Lohr JM, Bonge D, et al. A large sample empirical typology of male spouse abusers and its relationship to dimensions of abuse. Violence Vict 1996; 11(4):277–292.

26. Walker L. The battered woman. New York: Harper and Row; 1979.

27. Walker L. The battered women's syndrome study. In: Finkelhor D, Gelles R, Hotaling G, et al., eds. The dark side of families. Beverley Hills, CA: Sage; 1983.

28. Walker L. Violence against women: implications for mental health policy. In: Walker L, ed. Women and mental health policy. Beverley Hills, CA: Sage; 1984:197–206.

29. Gondolf EW. Reassault at 30-months after batterer program intake. Int J Offender Ther Comp Criminol 2000; 44:111–128.

30. Romans SE, Poore MR, Martin JL. The perpetrators of domestic violence. Med J Australia 2000; 173:484–488.

31. Hamberger LK, Feuerbach SP, Borman RJ. Detecting the wife batterer. Med Aspects Hum Sex 1990; (September):32–39.

32. Bowker LH, Maurer L. The medical treatment of battered wives. Women Health 1987; 12:25–45.

33. Searight H. The Tarasoff Warning and the duty to protect: implications for family medicine. In: Hamberger L, Burge S, Graham A, et al., eds. Violence issues for health care educators and providers. Binghampton, NY: Haworth Maltreatment and Trauma Press; 1997:153–168.

34. Dobash RP, Dobash RE, Cavanagh K, et al. Confronting violent men. In: Hanmer J, Itzin C, eds. Home truths about domestic violence: feminist influences on policy and practice, a reader. London: Routledge; 2000:290–309.

35. Taft A. Lifting the lid on Pandora's Box: training family doctors in the detection and management of intimate partner abuse/domestic violence. Doctoral dissertation. Canberra: Australian National University; 2000.

36. Katsikas SL. Long-term effects of childhood maltreatment: an attachment theory perspective. Dissertation Abstracts International: Section B. The Sciences and Engineering 1996; 57(3B):2177.

37. Grotberg E. A guide to promoting resilience in children: strengthening the human spirit. The Hague: The Bernard van Leer Foundation; 1995.

38. Hegarty K, Gunn J, Chondros P, et al. Association between depression and abuse by partners of women attending general practice: descriptive, cross-sectional survey. BMJ 2004; 328:621–624.

39. Golding JM. Intimate partner violence as a risk factor for mental disorders: a meta-analysis. J Fam Violence 1999; 14(2):99–132.

40. Dubowitz H, Black MM, Kerr MA, et al. Type and timing of mothers' victimization: effects on mothers and children. Pediatrics 2001; 107:728–735.

41. Laing L. Children, young people and domestic violence. Issues Paper 2. Sydney: Australian Domestic and Family Violence Clearinghouse; 2000.

42. Kelly L. The interconnectedness of domestic violence and child abuse: challenges for research, policy and practice. In: Mullender A, Morley R, eds. Children living with domestic violence: putting men's abuse of women on the child care agenda. London: Whiting & Birch; 1994.

43. Ulman A, Straus MA. Violence by children against mothers in relation to violence between parents and corporal punishment by parents. J Comp Fam Stud 2003; 34:41–60.

44. Campbell JC. Risk assessment for intimate partner homicide. In: Pinard GF, Pagani L, eds. Clinical assessment of dangerousness: empirical contributions. New York: Cambridge University Press; 2000.

45. Ferris LE, Norton PG, Dunn EV, et al. Guidelines for managing domestic abuse when male and female partners are patients of the same physician. JAMA 1997; 278(10):851–857.

46. Sassetti M. Domestic violence. Primary Care 1993; 20(2):289–305.

47. Goldner V. Morality and multiplicity: perspectives on the treatment of violence in intimate life. J Marital Fam Ther 1999; 25(3/July):325–336.

48. Goldner V. Making room for both/and. Family Therapy Networker 1992; (March/April):55–61.

49. Gondolf EW. Assessing woman battering in mental health services. Thousand Oaks, CA: Sage; 1998.

50. James-Hanman D. Enhancing multiagency work. In: Hanmer J, Itzin C, eds. Home truths about domestic violence: feminist influences on policy and practice, a reader. London: Routledge; 2000:269–286.

51. Abbott WE. Poor recognition of domestic violence by health professionals. J Gender Stud 1999; 8:83–102.

52. Lupton C, North N, Khan P. What role for the general practitioner in child protection? Br J Gen Pract 2000; 50(461):977–981.

53. Laming L. The Victoria Climbie Inquiry. London: Stationary Office; 2003.

54. Sugg N, Inui T. Primary care physicians response to domestic violence: opening Pandora's Box. JAMA 1992; 267:3157–3160.

55. Davidson L, King V, Garcia J, et al. Reducing domestic violence. What works? Health Services. London: Home Office; 2000(January).

56. Webb EJS, Evans MR, Brooks R. The health of children in refuges for women victims of domestic violence: cross-sectional descriptive study. BMJ 2001; 323:210–213.

Chapter 10

Medico-legal issues: when women speak into silence

Jocelynne Scutt

States should condemn violence against women and should not invoke any custom, tradition or religious consideration to avoid their obligations with respect to its elimination.

United Nations Declaration on Violence Against Women

CHAPTER CONTENTS

POLICING WOMEN – THE POLICE ROLE IN AUDITORY SILENCING

On 7 April 2001, at about 9.25 pm in Longford, Tasmania, Australia, Sonja Anne Mercer was shot to death by Darren William Batchelor, the man with whom she had lived for some 13 years. The coroner found she had died on that day of gunshot wounds to the chest and abdomen intentionally inflicted on her by her partner, Darren Batchelor, who then took his own life. As she was shot and died, two police officers sat in a car parked down the street, away from her home. Only an hour before, Sonja Mercer had told police she was at risk, had been threatened with death, and feared for her life.[1] Why didn't they hear her?

On 6 April, Ms Mercer told police, Darren 'went off' and had beaten her. He was, she said, 'a real sick bastard'. She was covered in bruises and it was on that night that she contemplated going to the police. This step was triggered by her finding a note written by Darren Batchelor and addressed to their 11-year-old son, Warren. Darren wrote that he was going to kill Sonja Mercer and himself, and that Warren had to go to live with his grandparents. Darren's note added his rationale: that he 'had to' kill Sonja and himself because she 'was a slut' and had 'been with someone else'.

On 7 April, a friend, Sherie Gill, took Sonja Mercer to Launceston Police Headquarters, where Sonja told police she believed Darren was going to shoot her and himself, explaining about the note, which she had destroyed as soon as she read it. She asked the police to find out the whereabouts of her son, which they did whilst looking up the register for firearms owned or possessed by Darren Batchelor. After checking, Constable Jones, who took Sonja Mercer's statement, returned to say that Warren was with friends, and that Darren had arrived at Police Headquarters when his father told him Sonja was there.

At around 8.45 pm, five people set out from the police station for Sonja's property to collect toiletries and clothes for Sonja, and to search for the firearms: Constable Geappen, a uniformed police woman, a refuge worker, Sonja, and Sherie Gill. Before they left, police told Sonja and Sherie that Darren Batchelor was still at the station and would not be leaving. In turn, police told Darren that the party was going to the property for the firearms and items for Sonja. Contrary to their advice, police then let Darren go.

At 9.10 pm Sonja and her escorts arrived at the house and went in, the police collecting two guns, wrapping them in a plastic garbage bag, and taking them away to the car. Sonja and Tanya, the refuge worker, packed what she was taking in bags. The police returned to ask whether there was another gun, because three were registered in Darren Batchelor's name. Not finding the third, they returned to their car, leaving Sonja, Tanya, and Sherie alone.

Whilst Sonja went into the kitchen, Sherie collected a bag Sonja had left in the hallway, and made ready to leave. Sherie recalled:

> I then heard one gun shot, and I heard Sonja moan and I think I heard glass shatter. I dropped the bag, turned around and ran. Before I was out of the house I heard another shot. I fell over outside and heard another shot and another shot either just before or just after I got into the police

car. Tanya was already in the backseat of the police car and I got in and the police woman was driving and she took off. I told the police as I got in the car that 'he shot her' meaning Sonja had been shot. I told the police that I heard glass breaking and I heard Sonja moan. Constable Geappen was trying to get through on the radio but had difficulty because there were others on the channel. Finally he told them that there had been a domestic incident. We waited on the side of the road for other police to arrive. We stayed in the back of the car for a while until we were eventually taken to Longford Police Station. I kept telling the police that I wanted to get away from the area as I was concerned that Darren was going to come after me.

The coroner found that there was a 'gross failure by Police to properly deal with this matter':

- The deceased Mercer was at Police Headquarters to complain of an assault committed upon her only the night before by the deceased Batchelor.
- Police, that is Constables Jones and Geappen, were also made aware of the death threat contained in the note made by the deceased Batchelor that very day.
- Those officers were also aware that the deceased Mercer believed that she required the protection of a Domestic Restraint Order and the information provided to those officers, properly considered, should have led them to the conclusion that this was the case.
- They were also aware that the deceased Batchelor was in possession of firearms, and had the means thereby to carry out his threat.
- The deceased Batchelor was also at Police Headquarters at the time, in response to having been alerted to the deceased's Mercer's presence there and was showing concern about it and appeared upset.
- It would have been simple, and certainly the appropriate thing to do, to arrest him in order to facilitate the making of a Restraint Order. Instead Constable Geappen, with the tacit approval of his superior Sergeant Hill, believed he had established such a rapport with Batchelor that he could trust him to be left at liberty.
- Arrest and detention would have been in accordance with the pro-charge, pro-arrest Police policy in place at the time.
- Instead, not only was he allowed his liberty, but was informed by Constable Geappen of Police plans to take the deceased Mercer to the family home to collect her personal belongings and to seize his firearms.
- He was thereby provided with both information and opportunity which would enable him to do precisely that which he had threatened, and which, indeed he ultimately and tragically did.
- Once it was discovered that there were 2 guns only instead of the 3 registered, police should have immediately evacuated everyone from the scene.

In 1983, a major study of 312 Australian families confirmed the police approach, which was not to attend 'domestics' or, if attending, to advise the wife that 'there was nothing they could do', 'it's just a domestic' or 'it's a civil, not a criminal, matter'.[2] Yet rather than require police to deal with criminal assault at home through the criminal justice process, civil injunctions were introduced in every jurisdiction whereby the battered woman could obtain an order that her husband or partner not beat her again. These orders decriminalized acts of violence against women which, if inflicted on strangers, would have been regarded as criminal assaults, unlawful wounding, or grievous bodily harm.

CHANGING LAWS, CHANGING CUSTOMS?

In the nineteenth century, the law not only condoned violence against women on the home ground, but saw it as 'husband right' (see Chapter 2). Judges declared this in their own words, or by adopting the words of earlier judges, earlier courts. A man was entitled to beat his wife, although 'not in a violent or cruel manner', and had a right to detain his wife, if she was on her way out of the house to spend 'his' money on clothes and fripperies.[2] By the end of the nineteenth century, the law formally recognized wife assault as criminal.

As for sexual violence, despite women's continued activism, it took one hundred years for marital rape to be outlawed by legislatures. In 1975 Sweden made it a crime.[3] In 1976, in a major overhaul of rape laws, Michigan in the USA legislated against marital rape when the parties were living separately and apart.[4] That same year, the South Australian parliament similarly passed a new rape 'code', including a marital rape provision. The bill originally made rape in marriage a crime, without distinguishing it from rape by a stranger. However, it was amended so that rape in marriage was unlawful only if:

- the parties were living separately and apart; or
- the rape involved 'violence';
- the rape involved 'unnatural acts'.[5]

This illustrates a confusion about rape and other forms of sexual violence, for rape in itself is violence. During the 1980s, most Australian states, Aotearoa/New Zealand, Canada, and some states in the USA introduced reforms, extending rape laws to cover marital rape in the same way as they applied to rape by a stranger. In the UK it took a decision of the English House of Lords in the 1990s to recognize rape in marriage as a crime, and the Australian High Court upheld state marital rape laws later in the decade.[6]

Despite protestations of men's groups, law societies, and many lawyers that making rape in marriage a crime would 'open the floodgates' so that numerous women would come forward to police with complaints about their husbands' sexual assaults, few women have, in fact, had the advantage of rape in marriage provisions. Few prosecutions of husbands for raping their wives have been undertaken by prosecuting authorities.[7,8]

Women had hoped that changing the law would bring about positive change, so that crimes on the domestic hearth would be taken seriously, with crimes committed by husbands at home being prosecuted, and courts recognizing the importance of applying laws women had struggled so long to bring into being through the parliamentary process. However, this did not reckon with the reluctance of police to deal with criminal assault at home, nor with the attitudes of judges and magistrates, most of whom were husbands with their own opinions about 'what wives should do' and 'what rights women-as-wives should or should not have'.

Customs underpinning marriage, which along with traditional laws saw the man as the head of the household, having rights and privileges denied to women generally and women-as-wives in particular, have a persuasive power. That power extends to all parts of the legal system despite its duty to ensure that women, married or not, are free from violence, and that men, married to their targets/victims or not, ought to be prosecuted when breaching the law. Thus, the principal changes to laws relating to wife beating, along with those applicable to wife rape, were bound to be subverted by custom. This was predictable, particularly where no educational programmes were instituted for the judiciary, lawyers, and police, ensuring that they at least had some possibility of having their minds opened to the spirit and meaning of the law reforms, and the principle that women were no longer the property of their husbands.

Although laws that subordinated woman's voice, identity, and person to her husband or father are now seen as archaic in Aotearoa/New Zealand, Australia, Canada, the UK, the USA, and other countries with a legal system derived from Britain, their impact remains. Laws arise out of customs, and laws beget customs. A change in the law does not bring about an immediate change in customs, because customs are embedded in inequalities between women and men at a practical level. This societal duality of laws arising from, and reinforcing customs, and customs lying at the heart of, and underpinning laws, means that in the short term, at least, practice wins out over theory.

DECRIMINALIZING THE CRIMINAL, LEGITIMATING THE ASSAULT

In the UK, USA, Canada, Aotearoa/New Zealand, and Australia, throughout the twentieth century, police spoke with one voice, across boundaries of nations and distance. When faced with complaints by women, children, or neighbours that husbands were beating and abusing their wives, police said they had no power to intervene in 'domestic violence', that it was for the woman to take action, independently, through the courts, not for them.

What police said was, however, not so. Through legislation and case law developing from the end of the nineteenth century, police had both the power and the duty to take action. Yet this did not shift the customary focus of adhering to the seventeenth-century notion that a man's home is his castle,[9] so that he could do what he liked in it – including beating wife and children, though not the dogs.[10]

The role of health professionals as expert witnesses can be crucial in the criminal justice process. But their contribution is dependent upon police prosecuting crimes of intimate partner violence. Evidence of criminal injury is irrelevant, unless criminal charges are laid.

If a police officer has a reasonable belief that a serious crime is occurring or has occurred, whether or not on private property, the police officer has a right (and duty) to arrest the perpetrator. Yet police said that if they were called to 'a domestic', whatever the sounds of violence within, if a man came to the door refusing them entry, they had no right to enter. The idea that a wife had no ownership in the property and no right to admit officers stopped them. Abused women and women's organizations accepted police lacked power. This was a mistake.

Lobbying of governments aimed at gaining laws to enable women to take civil action against their violent husbands rather than having police do their job, so that health professionals could, in turn, do theirs. Courts would grant orders saying the husband was not to approach or come near their wives' places of work or homes. A civil remedy was sought, rather than police extending criminal law rights to abused women.

The difference is crucial. In criminal law, police take, by investigation, arrest, and summonsing, to court the person they reasonably believe to have committed the crime. The state (acting through police, Director of Public Prosecutions (DPP), or District Attorney (DA)) initiates legal action against the person who has committed a serious assault, unlawful wounding, or grievous bodily harm. With 'simple assault' – no wounding, bruising, or broken skin, the person assaulted must initiate action, except where age, frailty, or other impediment prevents them from doing so. Women having a well-founded fear of abusive husbands should fall into this category.[2]

Civil law covers private legal actions – actions initiated by one individual against another. Responsibility falls upon the person seeking justice, to apply to a court through an application or a writ for damages, monetary compensation for bodily and/or psychological injury. The state is not involved, and bears no responsibility. However, if the woman wants the violence to stop, and protection against it, civil action is not what is needed.

Legislation framed for wife–husband situations was introduced to speed up the process of obtaining a court order – 'Apprehended Violence Orders' (AVOs), 'Restraining Order' or 'Restraint Orders', 'Non-Molestation Orders', 'Protective Orders', Intervention Orders' – to restrain the husband from physically interfering with the wife's bodily integrity.[11]

To obtain an order, the woman must prove, on the balance of probabilities, not only a physical threat or beating, but also fear or apprehension of future attack. If the court accepts that her fear or apprehension is real, the woman is entitled to the order. However, this depends upon the evidence she brings to court, and how well she conveys her fear. In turn, all this depends upon how the court 'sees' the evidence, listens, and hears – and the case has to be in court in the first place. This is dependent upon the woman's knowledge of the system, the readiness of the system to explain itself, and the attitude of court officials. By providing a report and giving evidence, health professionals can help. But they, too, need to know the woman's rights, their role, and the court process. A temporary order can be issued ex parte (without husband or partner being present), for say two weeks, a month, or three months, then a full hearing is held, with both parties present, and evidence of violence and threats – medical reports, photographs, torn clothing. The applicant answers questions from the court, the abuser's lawyer, or the abuser.[12] The judge or magistrate hearing the application is crucial. Some courts recognize the trauma, some are oblivious.

On breach of an order, the abuser can be arrested for 'contempt' of court. Police pursue only a small percentage.[13] Some courts take breaches seriously. Others do not, commenting sympathetically about 'matrimonial difficulties'.[2,13,14] This supports police notions that criminal assault at home is outside the criminal justice system. Breach for 'contempt of court' elevates the dignity of the court over women's bodily integrity. Contempt of court is worthy of prosecution; assaults supporting the issue of the original order are not.

Thirty years have seen little real change. In 2004 Law Reform Commissioner Judith Peirce said:

> There is a belief that intervention orders are not worth the paper they were written on, and there's truth in that . . . They can be effective in the short term, but not on an ongoing basis.[16]

These orders are a diversion from re-education and training of police in seeing and hearing the realities of home-based violence as criminal. They interfere with the recruitment of health professionals as expert witnesses. They also subvert the need for re-education and training of lawyers, magistrates, and judges for the same reasons.

In Duluth, USA, from the 1980s police were obligated to follow through on criminal charges. Although many jurisdictions sought to emulate this approach,[17] the culture of distinguishing 'family/domestic violence' from *real* crime, reinforced by the move to intervention orders, meant that not only were women deprived of their criminal law rights, but there was also no (or little) incentive for police, courts, and health professionals to re-educate themselves.

GOVERNMENT POLICY – IS ANYONE LISTENING?

Government initiatives have evolved through women's demands for the recognition that violence against women is a justice, health, and social issue, with economic implications for work and government services, including housing, hospital and medical, counselling, and social welfare. Amongst others, government initiatives include:

- Public housing, with a policy that a person with an intervention order should have priority.
- Community education and education for police, legal, and health professionals.[18]
- 'Zero tolerance' – legislative reform and policy directives that police **must** arrest abusers.
- Over-arching legislation covering all aspects of violence against women and service provision, as with the Violence Against Women Act 1998 (USA) and its precursor.

JUDGING WOMEN – DEAD AND ALIVE

Police and courts are linked: what police do, or fail to do, affects what courts do or do not do. What courts do, or fail to do, affects what police do or do not do. What both do, or do not do, dictates the parameters of health professionals' involvement in the legal system.

Educational programmes for police, to impart some comprehension about criminal assault at home and other domestic violence as 'real' crimes to be policed as crimes, will be subverted, or police will be frustrated in applying what they have learnt, if magistrates and judges remain uneducated. If lawyers are not educated in the criminality of violence by intimate partners (or by ex-intimate partners), they, too, will undermine police efforts at enforcing the law. An educated understanding for health workers – medical practitioners, psychologists, social workers, and others – as expert witnesses providing reports is also vital.

Health workers' expertise can be essential to ensuring effective outcomes through courts. Rather than being reluctant to give evidence, this needs to be recognized as essential to the job description. Courtrooms are 'foreign places' for most health professionals. However, the health sector must learn to present reports with authority. Training in presenting evidence is essential to the curriculum if health professionals take their work seriously. An assured health professional can change the courtroom dynamic. Barristers and solicitors are accustomed to dealing with women, if at all, as supplicants, victims/survivors and, too often, cowed litigants. If a professional woman of authority speaks, confident of her expertise, barristers and solicitors are generally nonplussed. It is more difficult for them to use tactics of bombast, hectoring, and scorn. The courtroom may be daunting. However, health professionals' responsibility is to ensure that the information they hold is presented professionally. Their expertise, presented with authority, can have far-reaching effects on the court process, in the instant case and beyond.

Law is bound by precedent. Judges and lawyers look to past decisions as the rationale for present outcomes. Seventeenth- and eighteenth-century case law continues to be invoked against women seeking justice, right up to the highest courts. This, in turn, influences police practices, impacting on the role of health professionals at court. Apart from individual and police-culture prejudices, police anticipate barriers to successful prosecution.

Barriers exist in the substantive law, say, the notion that a woman should endure at least one beating to obtain an intervention or non-molestation order; then the order must be breached, before action is taken to arrest the husband/partner. This notion is founded (probably unconsciously) in case law of the eighteenth century. So, too, barriers exist in the way laws are interpreted, along with rulings that keep crucial evidence out of the courtroom, meaning the jury never hears it.[19]

Health professionals need to be wary of imposing their perspectives on victims/survivors, just as police and lawyers need to remember this. Women can be 'talked out' of giving evidence against their partners, or persuaded that their partners do not need arresting. Ironically, where police (and courts) complain that women refuse to give evidence or 'change their minds' about partners being prosecuted, their own (in)action or pressure can be the cause.[2,20] This is compounded by lawyers and magistrates advising female clients and litigants to 'make up' with their partners. Health professionals should not fall into this trap.[2]

When professional assistance fails, women can be forced into 'self-help' or self-defence, bringing them into court on murder charges. Although both a death and murder trial could have been avoided by competent health, police, and court intervention, the law then treats the abused woman harshly.

Seventeenth-century women who killed their husbands were guilty of petit treason (killing the head of the household equated them with a subject who killed the king). Men killing their wives were guilty of murder only. This differential survives in the disparate application of provocation and self-defence laws, which in their interpretation and application favour men over women. Hence, the provocation 'defence' extends to men where a woman says she is leaving (and he ends her life), or where the woman is a 'nagger' (and he kills her), whilst women who kill husbands in defence of their own lives are more likely to be seen as premeditated murderers than killing in self-defence.[2,7]

In both situations, health professionals' reports can be crucial. Medical reports are often elliptical or do not include clear statements of what women have said. Reports refer to 'domestic upset', 'arguments', or 'domestic differences', when women describe husbands engaging in vaginal or anal rape. Clear and accurate reports of injuries could properly support criminal prosecutions.

SUPPORTING OR DENYING WOMEN'S VOICES?

Law reforms are likely to be problematic. Two examples are:

- mandatory reporting by medical practitioners, nurses, and other health professionals where they become aware, or suspect, that injuries result from criminal assault at home or other forms of domestic violence; and
- repealing the rule that a married woman cannot give evidence against her husband.

Both raise questions of autonomy and agency, neither of which can be isolated from state responsibility. Too often responsibility is laid on women in the name of 'giving her control' in circumstances where 'control' misapprehends the situation. If a house is burgled or someone attacked in the street, we do not say they are robbed of agency and autonomy if police prosecute robber or attacker. If the police failed to do so, or left it up to the home-owner or street-attack victim, police would be (rightly) accused of neglecting their duty. Yet there is a tendency to demand that women victims/survivors should shoulder the responsibility of 'deciding' whether or not a police prosecution goes ahead. In no other area of the law is such a responsibility cast upon the crime victim. In serious assaults, the police duty is to prosecute. Intimate partner abuse (IPA) is a prime case where circumstances also require that duty in 'simple' assaults. This does not mean that women's autonomy or agency is removed. It means that the law is applied as women have a right to demand, police shouldering a burden that should not fall upon victims/survivors in the first place.

The plan for mandatory reporting seemed to spring from the best of intentions: antenatal nurses whose patients were most obviously victims of intimate violence wanted a law that would be on their side so they could stop waiting and start acting.[21–24] This is not a new idea, for under common law a person who conceals a serious crime (felony) can be prosecuted for misprision of felony.[25] On the one hand, mandatory reporting by health professionals is not out of step with the general law, so why is existing law not applied? On the other hand, the 'intimate' aspect of criminal assault at home (domestic violence) is seen as taking it out of the realm of gangland woundings or attacks of a generally non-intimate nature, where power differentials intrinsic to husband–wife relationships are absent. Arguments against mandatory reporting include that:

- confidentiality of health professional and client or patient are breached;
- client or patient's agency and autonomy are compromised;
- services will not match rising expectations;
- holding out mandatory reporting as an 'answer' wrongly inflates the value of the requirement, simultaneously inflating expectations of patients or clients;
- victims/survivors may be deterred from seeking help, endangering their lives or health;
- more violence may be promoted by precipitating retaliatory action against victims/survivors whose visits to health professionals result in reports.

Research exploring whether or not women agree with mandatory reporting laws is not decisive. Mandatory reporting is controversial among clinicians, patients, and domestic violence prevention advocates. Supporters argue that it will facilitate prosecution of batterers and encourage health care professionals to identify domestic violence and improve data collection.

Encouraging health care professionals to identify IPA is important, because often health professionals do not do so, shielding themselves from the reality of their patients' lives.[26] On the other hand, should the education of health care workers take precedence over their clients' and patients' privacy?

The research shows that women who are contemporaneously victims of violence are often more reluctant to see any advantage in mandatory reporting, while the more distant the violence is, the more likely women are to support mandatory reporting laws.[21,22] This indicates that immediate fear of the partner and lack of confidence in the ability of authorities to stop the violence are paramount. Introducing mandatory reporting laws is unfair to abused intimate partners, unless rights are extended to them simultaneously; the right to credibility, to have their fears of retaliation taken seriously, so that they can access full and proper protection from the partner's violence. Mandatory reporting laws are of no value if they expose women to more violence, or to a greater risk, because the criminal justice system does not follow through by policing and prosecuting the violence, or the social justice system fails to support and advance victim/survivors' right to live autonomously and free from violence and violator.

As to compelling wives to be witnesses, because the law saw wives as 'different' from other witnesses, women were robbed of legal status. Because the husband and wife were 'one', that one being the husband, the law denied women's rights as independent, autonomous human beings, downgrading women's rights all around. This manifested in the rule that a wife could not give evidence against her husband. Although depicted as preserving marriage and hence of benefit to both husbands and wives, the rule protected men's rights, so that criminally active husbands escaped being exposed by their wives' evidence. This meant, in turn, that recognizing a woman's right at law not to be assaulted by her husband was subverted by the rule that a wife could not be required to give evidence against him. Police taking no action could be 'excused' their failure of duty. However, not all violence is inflicted upon women in the secrecy of the home and, even if it is, others are sometimes present, including adult relatives, friends, and colleagues, and other evidence can be available from health professionals or neighbours. No legal rules prevent their giving evidence. Nonetheless, the woman's evidence may be genuinely crucial.[21,27]

From the 1980s onward, jurisdictions began removing the rule. However, women's 'right' not to give evidence against their husbands was transmuted into censure of women. Some women refusing through fear to give evidence were found in contempt of court and imprisoned. Yet some found the law reform supportive, for they could say that they had no choice, being bound by law to give evidence. The husband could not hold this against her. It was out of her hands.[28]

The contradiction stems from laws designed not to advance women's rights, but to promote men's rights and 'wife ownership'. Yet, when such laws are sought to be repealed or changed, there is a sense that women may be losing some advantage. Hence, any law reform struggles with having to overcome an historical sense embedded in the psyche. This says that whatever the truth of the lack of protection of women, or the lack of advancement of women's rights through the law, still, to change a law that may give some appearance of advantage (however unreal this appearance or perception is) may be to deprive women of that advantage.

The truth is, that if the rule excusing wives from giving evidence did not apply to anyone else, it cannot be said to rob women of 'agency' when the law is changed and women no longer have the 'advantage' (however spurious) of not being required to give evidence. Wives are simply placed in the position which applies to all other citizens. However, because women continue to live in a world of sex/gender discrimination, making wives 'the same as' all other citizens can result in inequality.

PROFESSIONAL RESPONSIBILITIES – RECORDING WOMEN'S WORDS

Whatever the rights and wrongs of mandatory reporting and laws that no longer give an 'option' to a wife to decline to give evidence against her husband, health professionals have a key role to play. If criminal assault at home and other IPA abuse is to be lessened and, ultimately, ended, victims/survivors of these crimes need to have focused care and attention by health professionals.

At all stages, health professionals' reports can be crucial. The need for accurate reporting and clarity about what women say is vital. Victims/survivors of IPA are, or can be, embarrassed by the circumstances of their injuries and the requirement of disclosure to obtain professional care. Their emotions and shock can impede the clarity of their statements. However, equally the listener is too often embarrassed and does not want to hear. Their own disposition can affect the way they hear women's words, or fail to hear them.

Stereotypical views of women as patients should not be allowed to intrude into the health professional's work. Myths as explanations for what women suffer should not be a part of the health professional's 'rulebook'. Nor should embarrassment stand in the way of professionalism, compassion, and care. As long as it does, victims/survivors will not receive required care and support from the closest end of the health spectrum, through to the legal system and the courts.

Awareness is also essential, of efforts engaged in so strenuously by some, of 'shutting women up' – the listeners or 'should be listeners' not wanting to hear, because it is too painful or onerous for them to listen, or embarrassing. It may be that the need to develop and nurture skills in this field is denied or unseen. Health professionals must be self-aware and professionally aware, to guard against this narrow approach, and be open both to listening and to hearing what women say.

For victims and survivors, speaking up is not the problem. For women seeking assistance from health professionals, lawyers, police, and courts, the obstacle is being heard. The problem lies with the professions and their (in)capacity to listen, to hear, to understand. For health professionals, this can be a failure on their part to hear what women say as victims/survivors of IPA, and a failure of police or courts to listen to what health professionals say as expert witnesses.

Women subjected to male violence know that the problem of women's silence is not oral, but aural. Women speak, but no one listens. No one hears. This aural failure is endemic. It exists at all levels of the legal system, to the highest reaches of the judiciary. It is replicated amongst other professionals – doctors, psychologists, psychiatrists, social workers, other health professionals, and priests and ministers of religion.[29]

That silencing through a refusal to listen or to hear remains, is obvious in policing of men who have beaten and threatened their partners, and in the judging of men who have made the threats real, by killing their wives. It remains in the policing and judging of women who, seeking to save their own lives, have been forced, through self-defence, to end the lives of the husbands who would kill them. Health professionals may pride themselves on being responsive to victims/survivors of violence and they may be more attuned to failures of others. They need also to see the defects in their own ways of looking and listening, becoming alert to the possibility that their auditory responses need reassessment.

Differences lie between law enforcement and delivery of health services. However, the history of both is the same: male functionaries, officials, and decision-makers dominate in the legal system. In the health professions, male dominance has been promoted, supported, and confirmed.[30–32]

Health professionals need to be professionally and self-aware, open to listening to, and hearing, women's words. Then, they can be positively professional, with an important impact on the way their professions work, the legal profession works, and the courts work. The health professions, the legal profession, and the courts are greatly in need of expert input, if they are to serve the interests of the community by playing their proper part in dealing effectively with criminal assault at home and its consequences.

REFERENCES

1. Record of Investigation into Death, Coronial Division, Magistrates Court of Tasmania, Coroners Act 1995 (Tasmania), Coroners Regulations 1996 (Tasmania), Coroner Peter Henric Wilson, 12 February 2004, at 1-2.
2. Scutt JA. Even in the best of homes: violence in the family. Carlton, Victoria: McCulloch Publishing; 1990.
3. Scutt JA. Consent in rape: the problem of the marriage contract. Monash Law Review 1977; 277–297.
4. Scutt JA. Reforming the law or rape: the Michigan example. Aust Law J 1976; 50:615–625.
5. Scutt JA. Consent in rape. Monash University Law Review; 1977:287.
6. Scutt JA. Women and the law: materials and commentary. Sydney: Law Book Company; 1990.
7. Royal Commission on Human Relationships, Canberra: Australian Government Printing Service; 1977.
8 Scutt JA, ed. Rape law reform. Canberra: Australian Institute of Criminology; 1980. *The 'floodgates' argument ironically indicated that men's groups, law societies, and lawyers putting this view accepted that rape in marriage was a problem – otherwise, there would be nothing to press open the floodgates.*
9. Semayne's case (1604) 5co. rep. 91a.
10. *When organisations such as the Royal Society for the Protection of Cruelty to Animals (RSPCA) were established, it was noted that they protected animals against harm from their owners, but there was no similar organization to protect children against harm from their parents – mainly fathers.*
11. *For example, in New South Wales they are termed 'AVOs' – Apprehended Violence Orders; in Tasmania the term is 'Restraint Order' (RO), in Missouri, USA, it is 'Protective Order'.*
12. *In some jurisdictions legislative action is being taken to deny the right of an abuser to cross-examine the victim/survivor. For example, the Victorian Law Reform Commission has recommended this in a report to the Attorney-General, August 2004.*
13. Wearing R. Report: monitoring the impact of the crimes (family violence) at 1987. Melbourne: LaTrobe University/Victoria Law Foundation; April 1992.
14. Murray SE. More than refuge: changing responses to domestic violence, Sydney: Allen and Unwin; 2003.
16. Munro I. Domestic violence: orders against abusers fail victims. Law and Justice Editor, Age; Monday, 22 March 2004: News 3.
17. *This has been common in Australia, particularly in the 1980s when (ironically) laws promoting intervention and non-molestation or domestic violence orders were being promoted, which downgraded the criminal element of the violence suffered by intimate partners, and transported this violence into the realm of the civil law.*
18. *In the Atherton Tablelands and Townsville in Queensland, in the 1990s, huge billboards carrying slogans decrying criminal assault at home were erected on the highway in to town and going out.*
19. *As an example, Dr Caroline Taylor of Ballarat University, Victoria, in her PhD thesis has critically explored decision-making by judges that keeps out DNA and other evidence in child sexual abuse in the family cases.*
20. *In Tasmania, at the 'Rape Law Reform Conference' in 1980, a 'training film' for police showed this graphically. The woman, who was crying out loudly for her husband to be 'taken away' by police who had attended at the home after she had been assaulted, was spoken to over an*

extensive period in the film, with police seeking to persuade her that she 'didn't really want to see her husband go to prison'. Despite her stating clearly the opposite, the pressure of police reiterating this over and over eventually wore her down. Scutt JA, ed. Rape law reform. Canberra: Australian Institute of Criminology; 1980.

21. Mooney DR, Rodriguez M. California healthcare workers and mandatory reporting of intimate violence. Hastings Women's Law Journal Winter 1996; 7:85.

22. Rodriguez MA, McLoughlin E, Gregory N, et al. Mandatory reporting of domestic violence injuries to the police: what do emergency department patients think? JAMA 2001; 283(5):580. *They report that between 1991 and 1994, four USA states – California, Colorado, Rhode Island, and Kentucky – 'passed various forms of mandatory reporting laws requiring healthcare professionals to report intimate partner violence to police. California has required reporting to police by clinicians since 1994, even if against the wishes of the patient/client.' Subsequently, further states have passed similar laws.*

23. Rodriquez MA, Sheldon WR, Rao N. Abused patients' attitudes about mandatory reporting of intimate partner abuse injuries to police. Women Health 2002; 25(2–3):135–147.

24. Hyman A, Schillinger D, Lo B. Mandating reporting of domestic violence: do they promote patient well-being? JAMA 1995; 273(22):1761. *In 1995, laws in 45 states and the District of Columbia mandated reports of injuries by weapons, crimes, violence, intentional acts, or abuse, with some reporting in cases of domestic violence.*

25. *In a classic misprision of felony, in a notorious case of the 1950s a gangster lying seriously wounded in a hospital in Melbourne refused to disclose the party who had shot him.*

26. The work of the Australian Medical Association highlighting this was cited in the High Court in Osland's case (1998) CLR 257.

27. Bachman R. Violence against women: national crime victimization survey. Bureau of Justice Statistics, US Department of Justice. Report NO. 94-0092-P; 1994. *In the USA, research confirms that victims/survivors are twice as likely to be injured during a crime if the offender is related to her and not a stranger.*

28. *This is often the case where witnesses give evidence against employers, workmates, or others with whom they are in a close relationship, personal or professional. They give evidence freely if summonsed or subpoenaed to court, because they have no choice but to obey the summons or subpoena.*

29. A pastoral report to the churches on sexual violence against women and children of the church community. Royal Women's Hospital, Carlton, Australia: CASA House, Centre Against Sexual Assault, Royal Women's Hospital; 1990.

30. Rich A. Of woman born: motherhood as experience, New York: Norton; 1986.

31. Spender D. The making and meaning of feminist knowledge. London: Women's Press; 1985.

32. O'Faolian J, Martines L, eds. Not in God's image: a history of women in Europe from the Greeks to the nineteenth century. New York: Harper & Row; 1973.

SECTION 3

Cultural diversity and intimate partner abuse

SECTION CONTENTS

Chapter 11

Cultural competence and intimate partner abuse: health care interventions

Michael A Rodríguez and George Saba

I didn't know. In my country there exists only sexual violence but violence between a couple doesn't exist because we are taught that that's a cross we have to bear with our husband.

Latina survivor of intimate partner violence[1]

INTRODUCTION

As national borders become more fluid and international migration increases, health care professionals strive to respond to the needs of their multicultural patient populations. This response has occurred at many levels, from the development of federal policies and national standards to the diversification of the health care workforce, and has included a call for all health professionals to become more culturally and linguistically competent.

At the same time, society has recognized the prevalence of intimate partner abuse (IPA). Health care professionals have also participated in a multilevel response to address the needs of those who experience IPA, through enacting legislation, developing clinical guidelines, and training clinicians from a variety of disciplines. Mounting an effective response to IPA, while being culturally competent, is particularly important because of the sensitivity needed between patients and clinicians. Frequently, the patient and the clinician hold different values and beliefs about the context and consequences of many issues, including abuse. In addition, the social stigmatization that often accompanies IPA represents a significant barrier to patients' ability to disclose IPA to their clinicians. Effective communication between patients and clinicians becomes paramount.

The purpose of this chapter is to explore cultural competence in the context of IPA as it relates to the patient, the clinician, the health care setting, and the health care workforce, and to present strategies to guide the development of cultural competency.

WHAT IS CULTURAL COMPETENCE?

While a variety of definitions of cultural competence have emerged,[2–4] this chapter will use the following:

Cultural competence

Cultural and linguistic competence is a set of congruent behaviours, attitudes, and policies that come together in a system, agency, or among professionals that enables effective work in cross-cultural situations. 'Competence' implies having the capacity to function effectively as an individual and an organization within the context of the cultural beliefs, behaviours, and needs presented by consumers and their communities.[5]

Becoming culturally competent begins with a solid grasp of the meaning of culture.

Culture

The thoughts, communications, actions, customs, beliefs, values, and institutions of racial, ethnic, religious, or social groups. Culture defines how health care information is received, how rights and protections are exercised, what is considered to be a health problem, how symptoms and concerns about the problem are expressed, who should provide treatment for the problem, and what type of treatment should be given.[5]

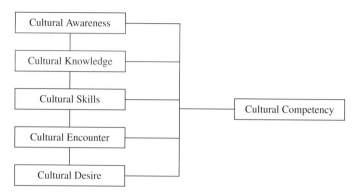

Figure 11.1   Adapted from Campinha-Bacote model of culturally competent care.[6]

Figure 11.1 describes a model that defines cultural competence as a continual process whereby a clinician strives to work effectively within the cultural context of patient, family, or community.[6]

Cultural awareness – becoming sensitive to the values and practices of patients' cultures. This process includes examining one's own cultural background and biases/prejudices toward other cultures.

Cultural knowledge – securing a foundation about the worldviews of different cultures. Here, for example, the clinician is able to obtain information about how IPA is generally defined within the culture.

Cultural skill – collecting relevant cultural data regarding patients' health histories and appraising cultural beliefs, values, and practices to determine the patient's perception of the problem, their needs, and possible solutions. In the case of IPA, cultural skill enables clinicians to learn systematically from their patients' perception of the situation and what they believe can and should be done about it.

Cultural encounter – engaging directly with patients of different backgrounds. Direct cultural encounters help clinicians to avoid stereotyping individuals within a cultural mould and to learn about intra-ethnic variation.

Cultural desire – motivating clinicians to become culturally competent. This caring is experienced by patients in a positive manner, as they value the fact that their clinician cares.

To become culturally competent, clinicians need to (a) become comfortable with differences; (b) acquire the ability to control and change false beliefs and assumptions; (c) respect and appreciate the values and beliefs of those who are different; (d) think flexibly; and (e) behave flexibly.[7]

These skills help clinicians avoid the tendency to learn a long list of culture-specific values and behaviours that may lead to stereotypes about groups and pay too little attention to the individual patient. While culture impacts health and health care, other factors are also influential (e.g. socioeconomic status, previous and current health status, history, geography, politics, migration patterns, language, and racism). Insufficient and incomplete training in cultural competence may lead health professionals to believe that culture accounts for all the variance they see in patients. If they concentrate only on issues of culture, they may miss significant arenas of influence that may provide more appropriate opportunities for care. For example, a clinician may assume that a migrant woman who has delayed reporting IPA did so because of culturally held beliefs about roles of women. However, unless the clinician realizes that this woman has limited geographic access to health care and that other non-migrant women in her neighbourhood also delay reporting IPA, the clinician may focus on cultural issues rather than improve patients' access to care. Overly focusing on cultural beliefs and values to the exclusion of other variables (e.g. social, economic, political) can lead clinicians to attribute people's behaviour as primarily relating to their membership in a particular subculture and foster 'blaming' the victim.[8]

CULTURAL ASPECTS OF IPA

The following examples illustrate the complexity of IPA within multicultural contexts.

Example 1

A 52-year-old woman was hospitalized with serious injuries after being beaten by her husband. Her 17-year-old son had called the police when he found his mother beaten and informed them that his father was the abuser. The son had been trying for years to protect his mother from frequent abuse by his father. The family was Filipino-American. The mother and son felt they could not previously involve the police for risk of embarrassment for the family. The father was a prominent man in the Filipino community. This episode of abuse was too severe for the son, and he decided to break the unspoken rule. The father was arrested and gaoled. While the mother was hospitalized, their extended family and many people in the community were outraged at the charges against the father. They blamed the mother and son for what had happened to her and ostracized them from the community. They told the mother and son that they were ungrateful for all that the father had done for them and had indeed brought shame onto themselves. They defended the father and took legal action to get him out of gaol. The son and the mother were left alone without support. The clinicians involved faced a complex set of problems interweaving cultural values and IPA.

Example 2

A woman, who had just delivered her first child three months previously, confided in her family physician that her husband had been physically abusive to her both throughout the pregnancy and since the birth. This East Indian woman had been reluctant to reveal the abuse because she worried about repercussions from her husband. The physician and the woman talked about the options, and the woman decided to let the physician report the abuse. The husband was arrested, and spent a few days in gaol but was returned home to the family after agreeing to anger management treatment and family therapy. During family therapy, the husband and wife discussed their relationship and the abuse. He admitted getting angry with her but refused to admit that he hit her. Every week, they both stated that things were getting better. Both their families still lived in India. His family was financially wealthy and powerful, hers less so. She reported that his family had made her family suffer for the reporting of the abuse. In conjoint meetings the wife said he no longer was either emotionally or physically abusive. However, meeting individually with the wife, she began to admit that he was still abusive, but would not say so in front of him. She wanted the therapist to meet with him alone and tell him to stop. She said he would listen to the therapist and would not listen to her. She also told the therapist not to say anything until she received final documentation that would allow her to become a citizen of the USA. Her husband threatened to divorce her and lie in order to prevent her eligibility for citizenship. The therapist found himself in a difficult situation fraught with cultural, economic, political, and therapeutic issues.

These examples highlight how cultural issues can emerge in IPA. Culture provides an agreed-upon set of beliefs and strategies to help explain the complex and uncertain experiences of life. When IPA occurs, culture can provide explanations and methods of coping while providing guidance for the roles all participants should play. Cultural belief systems about IPA can further define gender and family roles while also influencing disclosure.[1] For example, Yoshihama[9] interviewed 221 Japanese and Japanese-American women and found that 71% of the respondents reported that their Japanese background influenced their experiences with IPA. Japanese cultural beliefs about conflict avoidance, the value of endurance and collective family welfare, acceptance of male domination, and an aversion to seeking help were factors that influenced how they responded to the violence. On the other hand, research with African-American women suggested that they were less inclined to report abuse because they feared the police would mistreat the abuser; they did not want to perpetuate stereotypes about black men or women; and they felt it was their responsibility to keep their family together.[10–12] For some traditional Chinese women fear of losing custody of their children created a reluctance to disclose IPA.[13]

Furthermore, religious beliefs can influence a person's experience of IPA and their willingness to disclose. Jewish women may feel they should keep peace in the home and not bring shame upon the family. Christian women may feel that the scriptures require them to remain in the marriage regardless of what happens and 'turn the other cheek'. Buddhists may value perseverance, and feel that IPA is part of their fate and should be endured.[14,15]

Cultural gender norms can further influence how people define abuse. For example, Torres[16] found that 92% of Anglo-American women identified being punched, slapped, pushed, or having their hair pulled by a spouse as abusive. However, only 62% of Mexican-American women identified those behaviours as abusive. These participants emphasized the centrality of the family and male dominance as contributing ideologies to their definitions of abuse. Many of these cultural beliefs and values have a deep influence on societies, often reinforced by custom, tradition, and law. To varying degrees, some cultures have forced women into a subordinate role and treated them as less than equal to men. These roles can place women at greater risk for IPA if the society sanctions abusive behaviour towards women (e.g. marriage dowry deaths, bride price, female genital mutilation, honour crimes, distortion of religious scriptures to permit wife-beating, and lack of enforcement against husbands' assault and battery of their wives).[17–19]

While research is growing about the cultural aspects of IPA, the field is still in its early stages. It can be very tempting to latch onto a particular study and generalize about the larger cultural group associated with the sample. Differences exist within cultures, within generations, and within families. Moreover, gender inequality is being challenged as the primary factor determining domestic violence. Collins[20] strongly urges that we examine unique difficulties that women from different racial, ethnic, class, religious, immigrant status, and sexual orientation backgrounds face while concurrently exploring how power and control operate to oppress women from different backgrounds. Health professionals must be cautious, since more research is still needed to help them make decisions regarding considerable variations that exist in how people within a culture respond to dominant values. The clinician should consider that the best expert on the culture is the person who has come to see them. The patient will be the most able to identify how their cultural beliefs influence their gender roles; expectations in family roles; what constitutes abuse; and how willing they are to disclose, and why. Clinicians should familiarize themselves with general values about IPA in those particular cultures that their patients represent; however, they should then trust that those who experience the IPA can supply the best answers from their cultural lens. In that regard, the following questions can help guide the clinician to discover how culture and IPA intersect in the lives of their clients:

1. *The role of women.* Are they expected to be submissive, protective of their partners, silent, and accepting of partners' behaviour? Should they stay or leave the relationship if it is abusive?
2. *The abusive act.* What caused it? How could it have been prevented? Whose fault is it? How should the abused person respond? Should anyone be told about the abuse? If so, should this be within the family, the cultural community, and/or societal institutions (e.g. police, health care, clergy)?
3. *The abuser.* Should they be punished, forgiven, exposed, left, or asked to leave?
4. *The response to abuse.* How should family members and friends respond to the abuse? Should they hide it, deny it, or expose it? Should they take a primary role in attempting to heal the couple and/or correct the situation? Should they interact with institutions? Will those who report abuse be supported or ostracized from the community?
5. *Access to care.* How accessible are services (e.g. shelters, counsellors, legal aid, medical providers)? Are these services affordable? Do they provide necessary linguistic assistance? Are they staffed by culturally competent professionals? How responsive are they to the needs of the abused person?

6. *Trust*. Do the abused person and family members trust the broader societal institutions? Do they have suspicion, fear of discrimination, and/or concern about governmental involvement in their lives (e.g. deportation, loss of benefits)?

7. *Economics*. If the abused person wishes to leave the relationship, can he or she financially afford to do so?

While these domains exist for all people who experience IPA, the specific responses to such questions may be greatly influenced by the cultural and contextual realities for each relationship.

WHY CULTURAL COMPETENCY?

The demographic shift

Among many compelling reasons to embrace cultural competency is the need to work effectively with increasing ethnic diversity in most countries. For example, England has almost 6.4 million residents who are members of ethnic minority communities, constituting 12.5% of the English population.[21] In Australia, approximately one in four people is a first-generation immigrant, and 60% of Australian immigrants come from a non-English-speaking background.[22] This phenomenon of increasing ethnic diversity is even more visible in the United States. Ethnic minority populations have risen from 24 to 30% of the US population since 1990.[23,24]

The 2000 United States Census found that more than 46 million residents speak a language different from their primary care clinicians.[24] The demographic profile of clinicians, however, is not keeping up with the demographic changes of the population as a whole. For example, while the 2002 California population was 34.5% Latino, only 4% of nurses, 4% of physicians, and 6% of dentists in the state were Latino.[25] The different ethnic compositions of patient and clinician populations underscore the importance of obtaining the skills to enhance clinical effectiveness for multicultural populations.

The increasing diversity in language, religion, values, beliefs, and customs requires that health care professionals consider how to adapt to new communication processes with their patients. Culturally competent communication is important because lifestyle, care-seeking, pre-existing health status, and outcome preferences are integral to the patient–health professional relationship and are also related to cultural diversity.

The elimination of health care disparities

Many ethnic minorities experience a lower quality of health care than non-minorities, even when controlling for the patient's insurance status and income.[26] Stereotyping, biases, and uncertainty on the part of health care providers may contribute to ethnic disparities in health care. For example, patients may not understand their clinicians and may not adhere to recommended treatment.

In Australia, studies have shown ethnic disparities in knowledge, attitudes, and behaviour related to IPA. Non-English-speaking background individuals have less awareness that IPA is against the law; less awareness of the different forms of IPA and the serious consequences it can have; and more beliefs that IPA is 'a private matter to be dealt with by the family'.[27] Another report found that 'Aboriginal women are less likely to report family violence, particularly to the police, whom they often distrust. They are reluctant to use culturally inappropriate support services, and in remote communities they may not have access to culturally relevant services.'[28] (See Chapter 12.)

WHAT WE BRING TO THE WORK

Health care professionals

Not only do patients bring culturally influenced values, beliefs, and behaviours to clinical relationships, but so too do health professionals. They exist in their own culture which shapes their views of help-seeking, care-giving, and relationships. Framing IPA as a health issue has made it necessary for health professionals to examine their own feelings about abuse and violence. They must confront their own preconceived feelings about whether or not different cultural groups may be at risk for violence. This requires that we reflect on our own belief systems and values about health care in general, and about IPA in particular, to see how they impact our clinical decisions.

Personal model of abuse

Saba[29] studied family physicians and found that they enter relationships with patients having a well-developed model of healing that is very personal and shapes their clinical decisions and behaviours. In a similar way, health professionals may hold very personal beliefs and values about abuse. To elucidate one's own model of abuse, one can reflect on the questions in Box 11.1.[29]

Box 11.1   Personal model of abuse: questions for reflection[29]

What do I define as abuse? How do I define physical, emotional, sexual abuse?
What do I think is the cause of abuse?
What do I think are the effects of abuse on health?
What do I think about those who commit abuse?
What do I think about those who are abused?
How do I think about guilt, blame, and responsibility as they relate to abuse?
How do I feel about working with abusers?
How do I believe one treats abuse?
Have I had any personal experiences of abuse? If so, how do they affect my work?
*Do I believe clinicians should care for the abuser and the abused if they are
    within the same family?*
What do I believe about reporting abuse?
*What do I believe is my role in working with partners/families where abuse has
    occurred?*

Answering such questions can help health professionals begin to identify what beliefs, values, and assumptions affect their treatment of IPA. Cultural competence goes beyond mastery of a finite body of knowledge; it is a commitment to lifelong self-reflection and humility.[30] In this process, health professionals acknowledge and manage the power imbalances that exist between themselves and their patients and develop mutually respectful partnerships. Through humility, they can better avoid stereotyping patients and assess the cultural realities of each individual. One way to achieve humility is through a patient-focused interviewing style that encourages patients to share their own stories and priorities.

Health care institutions

In addition to health professionals' personal values, we must consider the assumptions upon which biomedical health care systems are based. Many of these systems may have a dramatic impact on patients who do not share the same culturally influenced assumptions. Understanding the cultural values of biomedical health care, practices, and expectations can provide a context for understanding the lack of cooperation between patients and health professionals who are culturally discordant.

Our health care systems are, in large part, based on values and assumptions that grew from Western European beliefs and practices. This biomedical set of health care beliefs views life as governed by a series of physical and chemical processes that can be studied and potentially controlled. It endorses many values such as: time is important, especially the health professionals' time; patients are seen by appointment only; health care is private; law mandates confidentiality; professionalism is impersonal; personal involvement is bad; families get in the way; visiting hours should be limited; health care is delivered during the working week; good patients will keep their appointments; good patients comply with treatment plans; the clinician knows best; providers prefer patients who can pay for services; and health care is a business.

Limitations of the biomedical health care system include: (a) restrictions on the knowledge considered to be 'relevant' to a particular disease; (b) limitations on how we elicit and present information to patients; (c) neglect of culturally relevant data which can impede the establishment of mutual trust and acceptance within some cultures; (d) inadequate exploration of patients' expectations and goals for treatment, which can decrease patient collaboration and cooperation. In contrast, the biopsychosocial framework explores health and illness within a vast network of interconnected subsystems (e.g. biosphere, nations, culture, subculture, community, family, individuals (intrapersonal behaviour, cognitions, emotions, organ systems, cells, and atoms)), and facilitates care within the context of human relationships. Adopting a biopsychosocial model provides a helpful framework for understanding the cultural context of patients and treating the multiple complex issues of IPA. Maintaining a broader perspective on providing culturally competent care can also direct attention to inner resources, values, intelligence, spirituality, and wisdom that is inherently present in all patients.[31]

STRATEGIES AND APPROACHES THAT GUIDE CULTURAL COMPETENCE

Several strategies can foster cultural competency in the care of IPA.

Individual strategies for cultural competence

One strategy includes asking patients the following questions:[32]

- What do you call your troubles?
- Why do you think your illness started?
- When did it begin?
- How severe is it?
- What do you fear the most about your illness?
- What are the major problems your illness has caused?
- What kind of treatment (or referrals) do you think you should receive?

When applied to adults receiving routine ambulatory care, the LEARN model improved cross-cultural communication and empathy, and patients became actively engaged in their health care.[33,34] The LEARN model includes:

- Listening to the patient's perspective;
- Explaining and sharing one's own perspective;
- Acknowledging differences and similarities between these two perspectives;
- Recommending a treatment plan;
- Negotiating a mutually agreed-on treatment plan.[35]

Health professionals should be cautious, however, in depending too rigidly on guidelines. Too frequently, we search for the body of cultural facts that once learned will improve our care. Cultural competence requires more than the application of protocols or acquiring the 'do's and don'ts' of a content-oriented approach to learning. A more process-oriented model goes beyond learning the informational content about cultural care. It appreciates that not all members of a gender, a family, or a culture ascribe to the same values that might be prevalent in the dominant society. It operates in a mutually safe and trusting relationship that requires attention to process. Creating a context for healing would require clinicians to transmit respect rather than dismissal of patients' views and overtly state that they want to know if patients disagree with anything they say. A process-oriented model would: (a) train health professionals to learn about the cultural backgrounds (e.g. history, economics, geography, migration patterns, and dominant societal values) common to the particular racial/ethnic populations that they serve; (b) assume that the patients/families are experts on their own culture; (c) explore how the patient/family has incorporated or reacted to the various cultural aspects of their background; and (d) explore if significant differences in values exist within the same family.

Members of many minority groups find that language barriers pose a significant problem in their efforts to access health care. When the health professional and the patient do not speak the same language it can lead to loss of important cultural information, misunderstanding of instruction, poorly shared decision-making, or even ethical compromises. IPA identification and intervention is difficult without the proper linguistic tools. Linguistic difficulties may lead to poor appointment attendance and result in decreased satisfaction with services.[36] The common use of family members as interpreters can contribute additional barriers and discourage disclosure when addressing IPA and sexual practices. Frequently, the younger generations of families who have immigrated are the first to acquire English proficiency; however, it is inappropriate to place children in the role of asking and interpreting information about abuse between their parents. To address these issues, the US has developed National Standards for linguistically appropriate services in health care, which include the use of certified translators and assuring competent interpretive services.[37] Box 11.2 presents specific guidelines for working with interpreters.

Box 11.2   Guidelines for working with interpreters

Use professionally trained interpreters.
Avoid using children, other relatives, or friends to interpret.
Meet with the interpreter prior to visit to share the agenda.
Treat the interpreter professionally and with respect.
Talk directly to the patient, not the interpreter.
Use words, not gestures, and avoid technical terms.
Speak slowly, one question at a time.
Check in frequently with the patient to assure understanding.
Maintain eye contact with the patient by sitting/standing next to interpreter and
   across from the patient.
Allow the interpreter to interrupt if needed.
Repeat phrases using different words, if the message is not understood.
Stop the session and talk outside with the interpreter to clarify any confusion
   or change plans.
Be alert to any discomfort the patient or interpreter may have with each other.
Meet with the interpreter afterwards to get their impressions of the visit.

Educational strategies for training clinicians (see Chapter 4)

Training in cultural competency is recommended to improve patient–clinician communication and to serve as one approach to help reduce ethnic health care disparities.[26] Training health professionals to adopt a biopsychosocial framework and implement a process-oriented approach requires educational methodologies that allow for reflection-on-action.[38] These methodologies allow health professionals to learn, apply what they know, and reflect on that application, all within a context of peer support. Three methodologies show promise in training health professionals to achieve cultural competence in the care of IPA.

Articulation of one's personal models

To foster the articulation of one's personal beliefs and assumptions, one needs a context for reflection. Within a small group of trusted colleagues, learners can reflect on what they hold important and share this with each other. This process of articulation can begin with reflection on questions such as those in Box 11.1.[29]

Live supervision

To teach and evaluate cultural competence, it helps to actually observe what occurs in visits. Live supervision allows a trainer to observe and intervene during a clinical encounter. The clinician trainee and patient meet in a treatment room while a supervisor (perhaps with other trainees) is behind a one-way mirror in an observation room. During the visit, the trainee and supervisor can communicate via a telephone hook-up between the two rooms and/or can consult behind the mirror about such complex issues as one's personal reaction to the abuse, identifying and dealing with cultural issues which influence a relationship, and cultural dilemmas related to reporting. These visits are videotaped for later review. Through live supervision, clinicians can learn in the moment how to be more effective.[39,40]

Practice-based learning

In this methodology, a group of colleagues form an ongoing forum to focus on patients from their practice. They select patients who present challenges and generate the clinical questions that, if answered, would improve their care. Once questions are generated, each member gathers information to provide answers. This may involve evidence-based literature searches, consulting experts, and/or interviewing the patient/family. Members share the information and develop a treatment plan. The primary clinician implements the plan and reports back on the progress of the treatment over time. This methodology allows clinicians to build on their own expertise and learn from other experts – the community, the literature, and the patients themselves. This ongoing adult learning within the same group can build trust and enhance training in the complex issues of culture and abuse.[41]

Institutional-level strategies

Mandating behaviour change at the legal, governmental, educational, and institutional levels can increase health professionals' opportunities to become more culturally competent. For example, organizations that accredit training programmes and health care facilities could require that health professionals receive education and demonstrate mastery of core cultural competencies.[42] Accrediting bodies could also evaluate health care organizations on a quality of care indicator related to providing linguistically and culturally appropriate health care services.[4,43]

Another institutional approach is to recruit a more culturally diverse group of students into health care-profession schools. Prior exposure to ethnically diverse minority groups and students has been shown to increase medical students' plans of working in ethnic minority communities.[44] In another study,[45] African-American and Latino physicians cared for significantly more African-American, Latino, and low-income patients than did other physicians. Retention of these clinicians in practice and academic faculty positions is critical.

SUMMARY

Health professionals face significant cultural challenges in caring for people who have experienced IPA. Western culture has only recently begun to accept IPA as a health issue. Health professionals may not even be aware of their own personal beliefs and values regarding IPA and those of the larger health care system until they are given the responsibility, mandate, and power to deal with it. These issues would be difficult to address even if all health professionals and patients reflected a homogeneous racial and ethnic cultural experience. However, given the recent changes in demographics in Western countries, a variety of cultural perspectives regarding IPA may exist in the therapeutic relationship. A culturally competent approach is central to providing patient-centred care that will be effective among increasingly diverse patient populations who experience IPA.

To increase our cultural competency in the care of IPA, we must foster a number of changes. Cultural competence is more than a 'finite set of skills'; it should become a core value of our professions and woven into our practice of health care. Cultural competence begins with health professionals' willingness to acknowledge their own cultural context and how it affects personal and professional perceptions and practices. At the paradigmatic level, adopting a biopsychosocial model of health care would expand our understanding, clinical care, and research into the multiple systems affecting our patients who have been abused.

At the educational level, we must develop proven models of training not only of front-line clinicians, but also of all professionals who interact with people experiencing IPA (e.g. administrators, police, lawyers, judges, researchers). Faculty development programmes need to train those who will effectively teach the curriculum. Innovative programmes require the creation of contexts in which health care professionals can explore their attitudes and behaviour and can be supervised during their clinical encounters. Significant administrative and policy support are needed to ensure that resources are available and that quality education occurs.

To discover how health care-system settings can provide better care, we must move beyond theory and rhetoric to find evidence-based approaches that can improve care. We do have sufficient evidence to consider some policy changes to reduce IPA and improve IPA prevention and detection: (a) training health care professionals in culturally competent IPA prevention and treatment; (b) establishing a role for community health care personnel within the clinical setting; (c) hiring a more culturally diverse workforce that matches the demographic profile of the served population; and (d) implementing and improving communication processes between health professionals and patients by hiring interpreters, using multilingual materials to disseminate health care information, and hiring a diverse staff. To facilitate the realization of these policies it is paramount that appropriate research be conducted to: (a) identify cultural barriers that prevent IPA detection; (b) measure and evaluate clinicians' performance; (c) create a quality indicator relevant to cultural competency; and (d) ascertain the effectiveness of multilingual health care providers versus the use of interpreters. While becoming culturally competent will require significant and ongoing personal, institutional, and policy changes, we will improve our care of those who experience IPA in our multicultural societies.

ACKNOWLEDGEMENT

The authors are indebted to Jennifer Toller, Manal Aboelata, Adriana Carrillo, and Natasha Castillo for providing background research, generously sharing their opinions, and assisting with editing of this manuscript.

REFERENCES

1. Bauer HM, Rodríguez MA, Quiroga SS, et al. Barriers to health care for abused Latina and Asian Immigrant Women. J Health Care Poor U 2000; 15(11): 33–44.
2. Cross T, Bazron B, Dennis K, et al. Towards a culturally competent system of care, Vol. I. Washington, DC: Georgetown University Child Development Center, CASSP Technical Assistance Center; 1989.
3. Adams DL, ed. Health issues for women of color: a cultural diversity perspective. Thousand Oaks, CA: Sage; 1995.
4. Davis K. Exploring the intersection between cultural competency and managed behavioral health care policy: implications for state and county mental health agencies. Alexandria, VA; National Technical Assistance Center for State Mental Health Planning: 1997.
5. Office of Minority Health. National standards on Culturally and Linguistically Appropriate Services (CLAS) in health care. Federal Register 2000; 65:247:80865–80879.
6. Campinha-Bacote J. A model and instrument for addressing cultural competence in health care. J Nurs Educ 1999; 38(5):203–207.
7. Pinderhughes E. Understanding race, ethnicity and power: the key to efficacy in clinical practice. New York: Free Press; 1989.
8. De La Cancela V. Minority AIDS prevention: moving beyond cultural perspectives towards sociopolitical empowerment. AIDS Educ Prev 1989; 1(2):141–153.
9. Yoshihama M. Reinterpreting strength and safety in a socio-cultural context: dynamics of domestic violence and experiences of women of Japanese descent. Child Youth Serv Rev 2000; 22:207–229.
10. Campbell, DW. Nursing care of African-American battered women: Afrocentric perspectives. AWHONNS Clin Issues Perinat Womens Health Nurs 1993; 4:407–415.
11. O'Herron MMR. Ending the abuse of the marriage fraud act. Georgetown Immigration Law J 1993; 7:549–568.
12. Robinson, MS. Battered women: an African American perspective. ABNF J 1991; 81–84.
13. Anderson MJ. License to abuse: the impact of conditional status on female immigrants. Yale Law J 1993; 102:1401–1430.
14. Buchbinder E, Eisikovits Z. Battered women's entrapment in shame: a phenomenological study. Am J Orthopsychiatry 2003; 73:355–366.
15. Macey M. Religion, male violence, and the control of women: Pakistani Muslim men in Bradford, UK. Gend Dev 1999; 7:48–55.
16. Torres S. A comparison of wife abuse between two cultures: perceptions, attitudes, nature, and extent. Issues Ment Health Nurs 1991; 15:16–23.
17. Niaz U. Violence against women in South Asian countries. Arch Women Ment Health 2003; 6:173–184.
18. Kulwicki AD. The practice of honor crimes: a glimpse of domestic violence in the Arab world. Issues Ment Health Nurs 2002; 23(1): 77–87.
19. Douki S, Nacef F, Belhadj A, et al. Violence against women in Arab and Islamic countries. Arch Women Ment Health 2003; 6:165–171.
20. Collins PH. The tie that binds: race, gender, and US violence. Ethnic Racial Stud 1998; 21:917–938.
21. UK National Statistics. 2001 Census data [accessed 25 July 2003]. Available from: http://www.statistics.gov.uk

22. Australian Bureau of the Census. Migration [accessed 18 July 2003]. Available from: http://www.abs.gov.au

23. US Bureau of the Census. US population projections, 2001–2005 [accessed 8 August 2003]. Available from: http://www.census.gov

24. US Bureau of the Census. 1990 and 2000 Census data [online] 2000 [accessed 8 August 2003]. Available from: http://www.census.gov

25. Dower C, McRee T, Grumbach K, et al. The practice of medicine in California: a profile of the physician workforce. San Francisco: UCSF Center for the Health Professions; 2001.

26. Smedley BD, Stith AY, Nelson AR. Unequal treatment: confronting racial and ethnic disparities in health care. Committee on Understanding and Eliminating Racial and Ethnic Disparities in Health Care, Board on Health Sciences Policy, Institute of Medicine. Washington, DC: National Academies Press; 2003.

27. South Western Sydney Area Health Service. Women's Health Program. Strengthening attitudes opposing domestic violence in culturally diverse communities: campaign report [accessed 25 July 2003]. Available from: http://www.swsahs.nsw.gov.au/whealth/Projects_Strength.asp

28. Queensland Domestic Violence Task Force. Beyond these walls. Brisbane: Government Printers; 1988.

29. Saba, GW. What do family physicians believe and value in their work? J Board Fam Pract 1999; 74(8):856–858.

30. Tervalon M, Murray-Garcia J. Cultural humility versus cultural competence: a critical distinction in defining physician training outcomes in multicultural education. J Health Care Poor U 1998; 9(2):117–125.

31. Saba GW, Karrer BM, Hardy KV. Minorities and family therapy. J Fam Psychother 1989; 6:1–16.

32. Kleinman A. Principles of cultural competence. Proceedings, national conference on cultural competence and women's health curricula in medical education. Washington, DC: US Department of Health and Human Services; 1998:11–15.

33. Bennet M. A developmental approach to training for intercultural sensitivity. Int J Intercult Rel 1986; 10(2):179–196.

34. Lajkowicz, C. Teaching cultural diversity for the workplace. J Nurs Educ 1993; 32(5):235–236.

35. Berlin EA, Fowkes WC. A teaching framework for cross-cultural health care: application in family practice. Western J Med 1983; 139:934–938.

36. Carrasquillo O, Orav EJ, Brennan TA, et al. Impact of language barriers on patient satisfaction in an emergency department. J Gen Intern Med 1999; 14:82–87.

37. US Department of Health and Human Services, OPHS Office of Minority Health. National Standards for Culturally and Linguistically Appropriate Services in Health Care. Washington, DC: March 2001.

38. Schon, D. The reflective practitioner. New York: Basic Books; 1983.

39. Saba, GW, Shore WB, Sommers PS, et al. Teaching a systems approach to family practice residents: the '2 on 2' curriculum. Families Systems Health 1996; 14(2):151–167.

40. Saba, GW. Live supervision: lessons learned from behind the mirror. Acad Med 1999; 74(8):856–858.

41. Saba GW, Vener M, Sommers PA. Collaborative practice-based learning model for residents and faculty. Acad Med 2000; 75(5):562.

42. Accreditation Council for Graduate Medical Education. Outcome project competencies [online] 2000 [accessed 15 August 2003]. Available from: http://www.acgme.org

43. National Center for Cultural Competence. Policy Brief 2. Linguistic competence in primary health care delivery systems: implications for policymakers [accessed 15 August 2003]. Available from: http://www.georgetown.edu/research/gucdc/nccc/ncccpolicy2.pdf

44. Pico E. First-year students' expectations of interacting with minority patients and colleagues. Acad Med 1992; 67:411–412.

45. Komaromy M, Grumbach K, Drake M, et al. The role of Black and Hispanic physicians in providing health care for underserved populations. N Engl J Med 1996; 334(20):1327–1328.

Chapter 12

Intimate partner abuse and Indigenous peoples

Judy Atkinson

I realized quite strongly whilst I was last out [in that community] that I have been kind of de-sensitized to a lot of stuff even though I saw it and saw it as wrong. When you sit back and think – this family just lost about eight people in a couple of months – pretty much all of them tragic or certainly preventable . . . from young, to not that old. In the meantime between a death and a funeral, members of the family are brutally injuring themselves and each other. When you look, you see the same patterns being played out everywhere. You hear stories about the reasons why the 17 year old committed suicide and you can't believe it. No good to hope that in 20 years it will all die down 'cause those babies are right there amongst it. I have an interesting reference point 'cause if on my mums side of the family, if between my grandfather passing away and at his funeral my sister had her jaw smashed by her partner and my mum's brother stabbed his cousin seriously the family would be pretty stunned to say the least. In [this town] it's not far off such an everyday thing that it's no real big deal . . . This is in a really small town. I really don't reckon any middle class urban professional person could go into that environment and be very useful.

This is work for people deeply connected and knowledgeable about what the hell is going on. I still struggle to put things into perspective and I really want to see some of these perpetrators punished. At the same time I have seen so-called perpetrators being created.

The words of a staff member of Gnibe, the College of Indigenous Australian Peoples at Southern Cross University, Australia, after a recent murder in a community where he had worked (personal communication December 2003).

CHAPTER CONTENTS

INTRODUCTION

Violence is a global public health problem. The World Health Organization (WHO) portrays Australia as a country with low levels of violence compared to most other countries.[1] The report, however, highlights clearly problems that arise when data are used as evidence for a country's well-being as a whole, without consideration of the situation of subjugated minority groups within that country. Australian statistics, implying that the country is comparatively non-violent in comparison with many other first-world countries, gives lie to the situation of Indigenous Australian peoples and the historical legacy of colonial domination across generations.

The Australian situation could be used by WHO as a template. WHO needs to review situations of minority populations in first-world countries in its attempt to understand issues of intrafamily and community violence. Attention to these issues and needs within populations that have been dominated across generations through slavery, conquest, or colonization is critical. Indigenous peoples have much to teach about the experiences of various forms of violence in colonization, its impacts across generations in manifestations of intrafamily and community violence, and their resilience in recovery from abuse.

The approach used in this chapter has been chosen to demonstrate the difference between cultural constructions governing Western research, which informs government policy development, and programme delivery to Indigenous peoples, and Indigenous research philosophy, theory, and practice. The difference is more than simply a focus on 'problems' as single issues unrelated to other life experiences, such as the title of this book suggests. The difference is in worldviews.[2] Indigenous worldviews recognize the interrelatedness of all things.[3] In orality, or the narrative transmission of life experiences through *stories*, we make sense of the world in which we live. Often our invaded world seems senseless. The chapter will first review the documented extent of violence within Aboriginal Australia. While there are similarities between the Indigenous nations of Australia, Aotearoa/New Zealand, the USA, and Canada, there are also differences. Attempts will be made to highlight the similarities. It will demonstrate outcomes of trauma across generations through statistics of family violence from recent Government inquiries. Even though these statistics are confined to Australia the reproduction of violent behaviours through trauma experiences in gender relationships, in generational layers, will be relevant to Indigenous peoples in other Western countries. The chapter will consider international Indigenous approaches to building on the strengths and resilience of people to be their own change agents, and healers.

A NEW PUBLIC HEALTH APPROACH

Public health approaches to violence are based on the premise that violent behaviours are learned, and their consequences can be prevented.[1] Prevention and critical intervention programmes will only be effective if researchers, policy-makers, health service providers, and workers in the field have an accurate description, analysis, and understanding of the contributing risk factors in intimate partner abuse (IPA). To understand the roots of IPA within colonized Indigenous groups in Australia and elsewhere, the historical, sociological, and psychological influences on individual, family, and community violence must be established. Many of the structural levels of domination and inappropriate policy practice that contribute to the incidence of IPA continue in political and government policy and practice today, implicitly linked with dominant societal and cultural constructions. Some social and cultural constructs create and nourish abusive behaviours and dysfunction within individuals, families, and communities. Colonization and subsequent government-directed service delivery have created situations where Indigenous women and children have been made particularly vulnerable.[4-6] IPA is predominately a male-against-female problem. Colonization imposed Victorian roles of male hierarchy and dominance, already encased in the culture of the colonizing groups. This subjugated Indigenous women and children and condoned the private use of violence. Western legal services have often responded to the needs of Indigenous women and children by labelling Indigenous male violence against them as 'cultural' – based in 'customary practice'. Furthermore, government consultation and service funding have privileged Indigenous male voices over Indigenous women.

The levels of IPA and violence are a recognized concern of Indigenous peoples internationally, evidenced by their attempts to influence government policy and service funding, conference presentations, reports, research, and Indigenous community organizational service provision.

Aboriginal Australians have spoken for, written about, and petitioned for a holistic approach to the needs of people who have experienced violence. IPA is one aspect of violence. The word 'experience' is used to acknowledge a person (including a child) who is violated by an act of violence, a person who commits an act of violence, and a person who sees or hears violence. Crotty names experience as feelings, perceptions, meanings, attitudes, functions, roles, and personal reactions to events.[7] Indigenous research approaches would consider experience as our greatest teacher, if we are able to listen and learn, as in *Dadirri*,[6,8] to the layers of learning, knowledge, and wisdom that can come from our experiences. We need to build on the courage, resilience, and resonance that enable us to survive and grow from painful experiences. *Resilience* refers to the ability to survive and move beyond distressful experiences. *Resonance* denotes growth and the ability to build nurturing respectful relationships.

THE DOCUMENTED EXTENT OF VIOLENCE IN ABORIGINAL AUSTRALIA

In 1990, an Australian Federal Minister said, 'Domestic or family violence among Aboriginal and Torres Strait Islander people has risen to levels which not only impair life, but also threaten the very existence of Indigenous people.'[9]

An Aboriginal leader, Professor Mick Dodson, believes that very few Aboriginal families are not struggling with the debilitating effects of trauma, despair, and damage resulting from their experiences of violence. Dodson referred to layered levels of violence among Aboriginal peoples, with domestic and sexual violence between adults having serious traumatizing effects. Even before children reach adulthood, they in turn become perpetrators of violence against members of their own families.[10]

To discuss IPA within Aboriginal Australia without providing context to the contributing factors would itself be a further causal factor in the increasing levels of violence under discussion. Suicide, self-harm, violence between family members, including IPA, child abuse, and abuse of the elderly, are all linked to political, social, and economic positioning, which is a legacy of colonization, resulting in dispossession of land, loss of cultural identities, and dysfunctional family relationships.

In 1988 it was estimated that IPA occurred in 90% of Aboriginal families living in the former government-controlled Aboriginal reserves or detainment camps in Queensland.[11] The reserves were established under the Aboriginal Protection and Prevention of the Sale of Opium Act 1897, through to 1939, amended to the Aborigines Protection Act – 1939 to 1979. This legislation was created in response to the trauma to Aboriginal lives resulting from the invasion of their countries, and resulted in a total system of control through government legislation and bureaucratic power vested in the Protector of Native Affairs and the State police acting as enforcers. The controls written into each new layer of amended legislation included head shaving, flogging, chained work gangs, and confinement in small iron sheds or watchhouses.[12] The Protector was the legal guardian of every Aboriginal child in the state under the age of 21 and could authorize marriage and adoption at the flick of a pen, and determine that a husband be sent to one place, his wife to another, and the children located in a dormitory at yet another location. The 'protection' legislation was supposed to create safety for people who had been traumatized. Instead it enforced subordination and dependency while refusing to provide basic essential services. It gave power to people who used their power abusively. It tore families apart. Feelings of frustration, fear, anxiety, anger, rage, hatred, and depression, as well as the essential need to suppress these feelings, became part of the day-to-day lived experience of Queensland Aboriginal peoples.[6] Distrust, suspicion, over-control, and jealousy were incubated when husbands and wives were separated, a jealousy which continues in extreme forms in actions of violence today. While alcohol was outlawed, the use of it was promoted in secret binge drinking. In the consequent brawling and release of emotions further violence and traumatization became an outcome. Such drinking, as a form of self-medication, enabled life to continue under the trauma-inducing conditions of a total system of control. But it promoted violence at its most base level – within the families and groups incarcerated. By 1959, the 'Protector' or Director of Native Affairs could proudly state that, 'We know the name, family history and living conditions of every Aboriginal in the State.'[12]

This 'total system of control', similar to prison environments, promoted violence in its subjugated populations. By 1990, in one community with a total female population of 133 over 15 years of age, 193 cases of injuries to women due to domestic violence were treated at the local medical centre over a 12-month period.[9] In 1999 it was documented that of the 76 domestic homicides committed in Queensland over the period 1993–98, 26 victims

(34%) and 36 offenders (47.3%) were Aboriginal or Torres Strait Islander, a group who make up less than 3% of the Queensland population.[13]

More recently an Australian government inquiry identified a frightening picture of an epidemic of adult and child violence.[14] While Aboriginal women account for 3% of the population, 50% of IPA incidents reported to the police involve Aboriginal women.

A recent compilation of data from the Australian Bureau of Crime Statistics revealed an over-representation of Aboriginal people in the criminal justice system.[15] Approximately 3400 per 100,000 Aboriginal and Torres Strait Islander men are alleged to be domestic violence assault offenders compared to 550 per 100,000 of the general population. Aboriginal men are 6.2 times more likely than non-Aboriginal men to be an offender of IPA.

Another report[16] found that:

- 68% of Aboriginal women surveyed said they had been abused as a child, and approximately 75% of those women said they were sexually assaulted as children.
- Approximately 68% of women abused as children said they still need counselling and support to deal with the abuse they had suffered as children.
- Over 73% disclosed that they were victims of abuse as adults. Of those women who were assaulted as adults, 42% had been sexually assaulted; 6% of those disclosed they were sexually assaulted by a relative; 79% were physically assaulted (including family/domestic violence); and at least 30% of those women said they suffered systems abuse.
- 61% of those women abused as adults said that they did not tell anyone what was going on at the time, and 58% of the women said that they still need support and counselling for the abuse.
- Furthermore, 80% of the women surveyed said that their experience of abuse was a factor in their offending, which included drug and criminal habits to avoid dealing with, or being unable to address, the abuse they had experienced as children.

THE ROOTS OF VIOLENCE

The WHO outlines an ecological model that is helpful in understanding the roots of violence in Indigenous communities.[1] This model identifies the multifaceted nature of violence, covering factors in child abuse, youth violence, IPA, and violence against the elderly. By focusing on individual, relationship, community, and societal layers, the model allows personal histories to be traced across generations. These personal histories are vital in understanding extended Indigenous families, or communities, which show multiple, transgenerational layers of violence experienced as trauma, escalating in cyclic patterns across generations.

Theories of traumatic stress reaction (TSR) and post-traumatic stress disorder (PTSD) have been applied to many recent disaster, catastrophe, tragedy, and criminal violence experiences of individuals and groups across the world, including to family survivors of homicidal attack and rape, domestic violence, and child physical and sexual abuse. Such theories are now being extended to encompass the experiences of Indigenous peoples and the impact of colonization.[17–20]

Figley defines TSR as the natural human consequences in response to experiences of disaster or tragedy where conscious and unconscious actions and behaviours are associated with dealing with the stresses and the period immediately afterwards.[21] The *Diagnostic and statistical manual of mental disorders* (DSM-IV) defines PTSD as the trauma which occurs when:

> The person experienced, witnessed, or was confronted with an event or events that involved actual or threatened death or serious injury, or threat to the physical integrity of self or others – and the person's response involved intense fear, helplessness or horror.[22]

The DSM-IV does not highlight the chronic, ongoing stress of particular situations or where the stressors are communal or collective, and cumulative over time. While inadequate as a diagnostic tool when considering warzone situations across generations, and where conditions and cumulative traumatic stress situations are ongoing, the DSM definition does, however, provide a starting point. Afghanistan and Palestine both demonstrate warzone situations across generations, because people have no other memory except the conditions of war and detainment where violence and death have become day-to-day 'normalized' experiences. Indigenous Australian former reserve compounds or detainment camps also demonstrated such situations. In many instances, the violence and death is internalized and the communities are now imploding. The experience for a child is of a war-zone.

Victims of violence, and those who work to provide meaningful responses to their needs, should not view traumatic symptoms as signs of personal weakness, mental illness, or criminal behaviour. The feelings and behaviours that come from traumatization are the natural and predictable reactions of normal people.[21,23–26] The traumatization is often collective, across whole communities, more particularly so for Indigenous peoples where family and community relationships are integral to cultural and spiritual identity. Such relationships have been fractured by government policies such as placing Aboriginal children in residential schools in Canada, and removing Aboriginal children from their families in Australia.

Although collective trauma does not have the same acute impact normally associated with trauma, it has distinct and, in many cases, longer-lasting repercussions. It seeps slowly and insidiously into the fabric and soul of relations and beliefs of people as community. The shock associated with the loss of self and community comes gradually. People, feeling bereaved, grieve for their loss of cultural surrounds, as well as for family and friends. Feeling victimized, the same people may also carry a deep rage at what has happened to them, but may be unable to express their anger at those they perceive to have violated their world and caused the death of their loved ones. They are not sure what to do, as often both their inner compass and their outer maps for what is considered 'proper' behaviour are lost.[27] Violence becomes transgenerational and words used to describe the individual and collective trauma provide intensity to its impacts: anxiety, rage, and depression; subjective feelings of loss; a sense of helplessness in the face of conditions over which there is no feeling of control; apathy; a retreat into dependency; a general loss of ego functions; and a numbness of spirit.[28]

Social order may also be destroyed. Simpson argues for the development of a greater understanding of community trauma and communal responses to trauma.[26] We must develop a greater understanding of the nature and effects of continuing and recursive violence and the interplay between multiple traumas. Most importantly, Simpson calls for recognition of the political context of trauma and its effects and the fact that structural violence, such as that inherent in oppressive systems, has potentially severe and continuing post-traumatic effects. It is this trauma that must be acknowledged in understanding the present escalating levels of violence in Aboriginal families and communities, more particularly IPA.

THE EFFECTS OF VIOLENCE ON BOTH VICTIMS AND THEIR FAMILIES

Physical assault represents only a segment of the total trauma experience of survivors of IPA. Such violence may include verbal harassment, psychological and emotional abuse, sexual assault, and economic deprivation. Injury to the psyche or spirit is primary in all these situations. Because of the relevancy of kinship bonds, the trauma of betrayal by other family members can often be overwhelming for Indigenous women.

Women who are being beaten may suffer severely impaired functioning in self-esteem, parenting, work functions, and social interactions. Generally they will have negative feelings about themselves and may view themselves as being of little worth, incompetent, and deserving of abuse. Often they become passive, despairing that they can do anything to change their situation, feeling unable to act on their own behalf, fatigued, and numb, and can do little more than achieve day-to-day survival.[5]

Violent behaviour becomes addictive. Some Indigenous men have explained how they feel more powerful, and have a release in tension when their feelings of low self-worth, fear, frustration, or jealousy are expressed in violent action. Violent assault has a spiralling effect on the abuser as well as the abused. Physical violence increases with the increased need for tension release and the increasing need to assert 'power over' as the one abused attempts to escape from the abusive situation. In fact, men who use violence to enforce dominance enter a revolving door of self-disempowerment. Australian research showed that 53% of the Indigenous men who died in prison or police cells were in custody for violent crime: 9% for homicide, 12% for assault, and 32% for sexual offences.[29] Most of these were crimes of IPA.

While Indigenous women say they want men who are violent to be dealt with by the criminal justice system, they also repeatedly say their men come out of gaol more brutalized than before incarceration.[11] Both Indigenous men and women have become locked into a dominant system which is providing few alternatives other than police action, prison sentences, or mental health pathologies for behaviours which are often an expression of physical, emotional, and psychic pain and trauma. Such approaches reinforce the notion that IPA is an individual problem and ignores the historical and socio-political impacts that are outside the control of the individual.

There is also an important link between violence against others and self-inflicted injury and suicide. For Indigenous people, the boundary between self and others is not as clearly defined as it is in Western society because of their collective rather than individualistic orientation. Amy Peters, who had scarred hands from smashing louvres, said, 'I reach a point where I can't get rid of anger any other way besides smashing things or getting stuck into somebody.'[30] Her brother Alwyn was on trial at that time for killing his partner.

Indigenous alcohol misuse is often cited as the cause of violent behaviours. Alcohol does not cause violence. However, alcohol (and other drug) misuse can contribute to, and result from, violent behaviours.[31] Evidence exists that Aboriginal women are drinking more because of their sense of betrayal at the abuse they are experiencing within their families.[6] Drug misuse becomes a coping mechanism, an adaptive way of dealing with trauma, stress, abandonment, anxiety, depression, or emotional distress and violence.[19] People who are traumatized may use drugs such as alcohol to cut off or block painful feelings. Feelings are suppressed or denied until a situation or event triggers an extreme outburst toward something or someone seemingly unrelated to the original trauma.

The use of alcohol or other drugs may also allow feelings of anger to be expressed. Anger is a normal human response to frustration, fear, or help-lessness.[32] It is an emotion that can be healthy or unhealthy and may move people out of feeling helpless, powerless, or frustrated. However, within some Indigenous families and communities anger is often expressed in violent actions. Such violence becomes learned behaviour. When we live in a violent society we learn to express ourselves through violence. Alcohol may or may not be a factor, and can be considered a tool through which such feelings and actions can be released.

It is clear that where the levels of violence and alcohol misuse have increased in Indigenous communities over the last twenty years, children are substantially affected and traumatized. One Aboriginal Australian Child Care Agency claims that 80% of the children they work with come from situations of IPA.[33] Such children sometimes have severe behavioural problems and lack social competence. Staff from an Aboriginal Australian women's shelter say that children coming into the shelter are already socialized to use violence as a form of expression and dominance.[33] Two- and three-year-olds will pick up a stick or a rock at the slightest provocation to use against other children.

Recent research shows clear links between adults who are victims and/or perpetrators of IPA, their childhood witnessing of, or experiencing, physical or sexual violence, and their perpetration of child sexual and physical abuse and neglect of their own children and others.[6,34] More importantly, such research shows that listening to the stories of people who have experienced violence and have rebuilt their lives provides us (and them) with a healing way forward. The use of *story* can inform a new public health model for an Indigenous healing response to the pain of violence that includes IPA.

STORIES OF PAIN

In 1998, towards the end of my PhD field research, I received a call from a doctor in the small town where I was living. He told me he had an Aboriginal woman in his surgery and he did not know what to do with her. The woman would not or could not speak to him, yet had come to the surgery clearly distressed. He asked if I would come down and see if I could be of any help.

When I walked into the surgery I was taken to a middle-aged Aboriginal woman sitting on a chair in a spare room of the surgery. Her two children sat silently in a corner watching her every move. She made no acknowledgement of my presence, so I sat on the floor close to her, allowing my hand to rest gently against her foot.

I told her my name and a small part of my family background, and commented that I had not seen her around town before, so I didn't know which family she was from. I was wondering, I said, if she had just moved here, or if she was passing through. After some long silence she told me she had just got off the train:

Me: *Oh, so you have come here to live.*
Woman: *No. I'm on my way home (to Sydney).*
Me: *Oh, and where have you been?*
Woman: *In Cairns.*
Me: *Oh I know Cairns, I lived there for some years. Do you have family there?*
Woman: *I was there for my daughter's funeral.*

My eyes filled with tears. My own son had just died in an accident some months previously, and I felt, as a mother, a deep connection to a woman who has had to bury her own child.

Me: *That must have been so hard? My son was killed last month and it is so hard* – (my voice faltered).

She looked at me for the first time since I had been in the room, and took my hand to rest it on her lap. After some silence she began to tell me her *story*: a long and painful *story* of multiple losses that bubbled out of her as if the telling had been waiting to be both told and heard.

She talked of the recent death of this child she had just buried as a result of IPA, the death of another daughter from IPA, the suicide of a daughter; the suicide of a son while he was in custody, all within the last five years, She spoke of her worry for her remaining son who was living in a rural north Queensland town, who was drinking too much and suicidal. She saw that I was crying, and she also began to cry, and then she told of her own childhood in the institution where she had been placed, and how she was indentured as a domestic at the age of 13 to a family where the men had used her as a sexual object; how she escaped to marry a white man, and had endured a marriage of 24 years during which all her seven children had seen her repeatedly beaten and abused, physically, sexually, emotionally, spiritually, and racially. She blamed herself for what had happened, and was happening to her children. She felt she had given them this legacy of violence. She was more particularly concerned for the two girls who were in the room with us, the 10-year-old and the 13-year-old (who was obviously pregnant). Two hours later, she stopped talking, looked at me, and in a clear strong voice said, 'Oh you're a good "doctor". I feel so much better now.'

Later the medical doctor asked, 'What did you do? There is such a change in her.' How could I explain that I had done nothing except listen, that the intuitive link which opened the door to her *story* was the feelings that connected us in the loss of a child. In my listening we had grieved together, and I was sustained and nurtured by her – her courage, her resilience, her deep and painful caring for her children, in spite of her own pain and painful experiences. We reached, even in our communal pain, a resonance, a healing communication, a language of the heart.

ANOTHER STORY

I had been working in relationship with a rural community where there was no doctor, and where the population of Aboriginal people, totalling 950, received their medical care from two registered nurses and a fortnightly visit by the Flying Doctor service. There had been a series of rapes of Aboriginal children and women, and at least seven deaths of women due to IPA over the period of years in which I came to know the people of this community. The legal system demonstrated no interest in pursuing the incidence of sexual or physical assaults except in the case of death where, under Queensland law, it was required. Police told me such behaviour was 'cultural'. In 1987, a small child had been raped and the elders in the community were in despair. They wanted the offender dealt with and removed from the community. They felt powerless, because they felt nobody would listen to their concerns. Some months after the rape of the child, one of the white registered nurses working in the community was raped, and this resulted in immediate action by the law enforcement agencies. A plane flew 2,500 kilometres from Brisbane, a person was arrested, and removed, and the nurse was also taken away from the community for health care. Three issues are important here:

1. The community saw action and, while very upset and ashamed that the nurse had been raped, also began to ask hard questions – why did they not receive similar treatment and/or legal responses to their needs?
2. There was general racist outrage by white public servants, which in the long term resulted in fortress-like hospital buildings being erected in communities to protect nursing staff.
3. More importantly, in discussion with the nurse some time later she told me that, before the rape, every day she would have a visit from a woman who had similar wounds that she sustained in the rape, and that she had treated the wounds while making judgements against the woman. She assumed the wounds had been caused while the woman had been intoxicated. She had never asked if the woman had been subject to sexual assault. She said that her experience had made her look deeply at her ethical practice as a nurse.

AN INDIGENOUS NEW PUBLIC HEALTH AND EDUCATIONAL APPROACH TO INDIGENOUS NEEDS

The above *stories* have been used to illustrate a number of points. Violence is not an individual issue. It has collective meaning with its roots in institutional racism encased in the histories of colonization, collective trauma, communal fracture, personally mediated distressed relationships, and internalized oppression.

Cultural barriers are encountered in the definition of health. The WHO's approach to health as the whole of life experience, defined as the emerging new public health model,[1] is more compatible with Indigenous concepts of health and well-being. However, Western medical approaches, and legal, social work practice, and educational approaches are continuing to be imposed on Indigenous peoples without acknowledgment of their inadequacy and potential for continuing harm.

The closest word for health within Aboriginal languages is *well-being*.[35] The word *punyu*, from the language of the Ngaringman of the Northern Territory, sometimes translated as *well-being*, highlights the fact that concepts and functions of health or *well-being* must be approached from an interdisciplinary and multidisciplinary practice. *Punyu* encompasses person and country and is associated with being strong, happy, knowledgeable, socially responsible (to take a care), beautiful, clean, and safe (both in the sense of being within the law/lore and in the sense of being cared for). It is further explained by Rose that '. . . when people and country are punyu the flow of energy keeps both strong, healthy and fruitful'.[36] *Punyu* and *well-being* connect people, place, and law into a whole, and is an '. . . achieved quality developed through relationships of mutual care'.[36] It is clear that health and law cannot be separated and are vital considerations in the development of policies and programmes of health service delivery around IPA.

Health services can be the first point of call for many Indigenous people who have experienced violence and they therefore need to be culturally accessible, culturally safe, and gender relevant to help alleviate some of the fear and shame that can be part of accessing such services. Cultural safety, initially the work of Irihapeti Ramsden in her work with health professionals in New Zealand, refers to: 'an environment that is spiritually, socially and emotionally safe, as well as physically safe for people: . . . It is about shared respect, shared meaning, shared knowledge and experience of learning together.'[37] Cultural safety 'extends beyond cultural awareness and cultural sensitivity. It empowers individuals and enables them to contribute to the achievement of positive outcomes. It encompasses a reflection of individual cultural identity and recognition of the impact of personal culture on professional practice.'[38]

'EDUCARING' AS A HEALTH AND HEALING RESPONSE TO IPA

Education is a vital consideration, which has largely been ignored in most evaluations of Indigenous family violence programmes. The word 'education' raises serious concerns for Indigenous peoples, however, bringing up memories of abusive Western educational approaches where the 'student' is forced to learn and perform with outcomes which are often unrelated to real community issues and needs. When Indigenous people talk about 'healing through education', and 'the educational processes in healing' they are giving value to the origin of the word 'education', from the Latin 'educare', to rear up, to nurture the children, to draw out from, to lead, to show the way.[39] 'Educaring' (my word), is used as an activity of experiential learning where the *teacher and the taught together create the teaching*. It is a process of drawing out the deeper knowledge which will show the way forward, and is the most important activity in working in the area of IPA.

Furthermore, when Indigenous peoples use the word 'healing' in the context of IPA, the concept is not given value within a Western paradigm. Warry provides an Aboriginal Canadian definition of healing that is particularly relevant in other Indigenous contexts[40]:

> Culture, identity, tradition, values, spirituality, healing, transformation, revitalization, self-determination, self-government: a spiral of ideas and actions constitute community healing. At the most basic level, when Aboriginal people speak of community healing they suggest that there are many individuals within their community who must heal themselves before they will be capable of contributing to the many tasks that lie ahead. They talk of finding ways to help support individuals who must heal deep wounds. This can only be accomplished if people are provided with opportunities for spiritual growth and cultural awareness. More generally, people must acquire new skills so that the capacity of their communities to engage in discussion, planning and control over their institutions is increased. There is a need to build supportive and healthy environments so that debate and dialogue can be conducted on the many complex issues that comprise self-government.

A healing educational approach is cross-disciplinary, integrating Indigenous cultural processes with a number of disciplines. These include health care practice and promotion, sociology, psychology, social sciences, Western biomedical and complementary medicines, law, history, and political sciences. Under an Indigenous definition the approach is holistic. Educational curricula should be blended into educational modalities which provide cognitive approaches, critical reflection and reflective practice, explication, and the insight that comes from experiential learning experiences. Such educational approaches would contain a training syllabus for the multi-skilling of all workers employed in the health, social sciences, violence prevention, and trauma recovery fields.

In 'educaring' approaches the emphasis must be on the relationship between historical and socio-political influences that result in social trauma and violent behaviour, and in particular how trauma and violence are transmitted, and consequently have inter- and transgenerational effects across societies and populations.

CONCLUSION

Educational, health, mental health, social services, welfare, and criminal justice strategies imposed on Indigenous communities to date have failed to impact significantly in improving outcomes for Indigenous children, and their families and communities. Indigenous children are sometimes immersed in families and communities that have been fractured across generations as a result of colonizing agendas. High levels of IPA are an indicator of that fracturing.

Support for innovative programmes to address the deprived and degenerating circumstances of Indigenous women and children and their families is urgently needed. Such support should promote resilience and resonance, a social learning model which draws on the strength of Indigenous worldviews of relatedness. Projects which focus on rebuilding community spirit and responsibility, with a particular emphasis on protecting and nurturing Indigenous children and their parents, are urgently needed.

Indigenous relationships are embedded in 'resonance', which builds relatedness and helps maintain healthy relationships.[39] We need to nurture the ability to support resilience and develop resonance in individuals, families, and communities by conducting specific educational activities reflecting holistic philosophies that integrate the body-mind-spirit. A community-based 'educaring' curriculum will centre on word language (which is spoken, written, or depicted in art form), body language (which is the ability to understand and respond to the body's messages), emotional language (which refers to the communication of feelings), and create and develop resonance. Resonance confirms well-being through healthy relationships with self, with others, within social worlds, and through professional practice.[32]

The conceptual development of building resilience and developing resonance is derived from an Indigenous educational approach which also reaffirms the new public health model supported by WHO and referred to previously. The model for 'educaring' involves developing mental, emotional, and spiritual health and well-being; the creation of healthier lifestyles; preventing child trauma; and increasing participation and inclusion in ongoing healing education. The most critical need we face is to strengthen our capacity to respond to issues of IPA, indeed all forms of violence, through education designed to address the needs of people 'at the coalface', and through participatory action and process evaluation research which shows evidence-based practice in policy development and service delivery.

REFERENCES

1. World Report on Violence and Health. Geneva: World Health Organization; 2002.
2. Yllo K. Political and methodological debates on wife abuse research. In Yllo K, Bograd M, eds. Feminist perspectives on wife abuse. Beverley Hills, CA: Sage; 1988:28–50.
3. Wilson S. Research as ceremony: articulating an indigenous research paradigm. Doctoral dissertation. Melbourne: Monash University; 2004.
4. Women's Business: Report of the Aboriginal Women's Task Force (Daylight-Johnstone). Canberra: Australian Government Printing Service; 1986.
5. Atkinson J. Aboriginal and Torres Strait Islander women and violence in the home: a strategy paper. Queensland: Women's Policy Branch Dept of the Premier Economic and Trade Development; 1992.
6. Atkinson J. Trauma trails, recreating song lines: the transgenerational effects of trauma in Indigenous Australia. Melbourne: Spinifex Press; 2002.
7. Crotty M. Phenomenology and nursing. South Melbourne: Churchill Livingstone; 1996.

8. Ungunmerr MR. Dadirri. In: Hendricks J, Hefferan G, eds. A spirituality of Catholic Aborigines and the struggle for justice. Brisbane: Aboriginal and Torres Strait Islander Apostolate Catholic Archdiocese of Brisbane; 1993:34–37.

9. Submission to the Royal Commission into Aboriginal Deaths in Custody. Cairns, North Queensland: Aboriginal Co-ordinating Council; 1990.

10. Dodson M. Violence dysfunction Aboriginality. Canberra: Australian National University Institute for Indigenous Australia; 2003.

11. Beyond These Walls. Task Force. Brisbane: Queensland Domestic Violence Task Force, Department of Family Services and Welfare Housing; 1988.

12. Kidd R. The way we civilise. St Lucia, Brisbane: University of Queensland Press; 1997.

13. Aboriginal and Torres Strait Islander Women's Task Force on Violence Report. Brisbane: Queensland Government; 1999.

14. Putting the picture together: inquiry into response by government agencies to complaints of family violence and child abuse in Aboriginal communities (Gordon). Perth: State Law Publisher; 2002.

15. Holistic community justice: a proposed response to Aboriginal family violence. New South Wales: Aboriginal Justice Advisory Council [online] 2001 [accessed November 2002]. Available from: http://www.lawlink.nsw.gov.au/ajac

16. Speak out speak strong: researching the needs of Aboriginal women in custody. New South Wales: Aboriginal Justice Advisory Council; 2001.

17. Danieli Y, ed. International handbook of multigenerational legacies of trauma. New York: Plenum Press; 1998.

18. Duran E, Duran B, Yellow Horse Brave Heart M, et al. Healing the American Indian soul wound, In: Danieli Y, ed. International handbook of multigenerational legacies of trauma. New York: Plenum Press; 1998:341–354.

19. Gagné M. The role of dependency and colonialism in generating trauma in first nations citizens: the James Bay Cree. In: Danieli Y, ed. International handbook of multigenerational legacies of trauma. New York: Plenum Press; 1998:355–372.

20. Raphael B, Swan P, Martinek N. Intergenerational aspects of trauma for Australian Aboriginal people. In: Danieli Y, ed. International handbook of multigenerational legacies of trauma. New York: Plenum Press; 1998:327–339.

21. Figley C. Trauma and it's wake, Vol. 1: The study and treatment of post-traumatic stress disorder. New York: Brunner/Mazel; 1985.

22. Diagnostic and statistical manual of mental disorders, 4th edn. Washington, DC: American Psychiatric Association; 1994.

23. Figley C. Trauma and it's wake, Vol. 2: Traumatic stress theory, research, and intervention. New York: Brunner/Mazel; 1986.

24. Ochberg FM. Post traumatic therapy and victims of violence. New York: Brunner/Mazel; 1988.

25. Silver SM. An inpatient program for post-traumatic stress disorder: context as treatment. In: Figley C, ed. Trauma and it's wake, Vol. 2: Traumatic stress theory, research and intervention. New York: Brunner/Mazel; 1986.

26. Simpson MA. Bitter waters: effects on children of the stresses of unrest and oppression. In: Wilson JP, Raphael B, eds. International handbook of traumatic stress syndromes. New York: Plenum Press; 1993.

27. Erikson K. Everything in its path. New York: Simon and Schuster; 1976.

28. Shkilnyk A. A poison stronger than love: the destruction of an Ojibwa community. New Haven: Yale University Press; 1985.

29. Royal Commission into Aboriginal Deaths in Custody. National Reports, Vols 1–5. Canberra: Australian Government Publishing Service; 1991.

30. Wilson P. Black death: white hands. Sydney: Allen and Unwin; 1982.

31. Herman J. Trauma and recovery. London: HarperCollins; 1992.

32. Wong B, McKeen J. Removing blocks to Resonance. IIHA Conference, Montreal; May 2004 [online]. Available from: http://www.pdseminars.com/us/articles/RemBlocksResonance.html

33. Atkinson J. Beyond violence: finding the dream (video and booklet). Canberra: National Domestic Violence Education Program, Office of the Status of Women; 1990.

34. Atkinson C. Review of programs and policies addressing family violence in Indigenous communities, Consultancy Report. Sydney: Human Rights and Equal Opportunity Commission; 2003.

35. Mobbs R. In sickness and health: the sociocultural context of Aboriginal well-being, illness and healing. In: Reid J, Trompf P, eds. The health of Aboriginal Australia. Sydney: Harcourt Brace Jovanovich; 1991:292–325.

36. Rose DB. Dingo makes us human: life and land in an Australian Aboriginal culture. Cambridge: Cambridge University Press; 2000.

37. Williams R. Cultural safety: what does it mean for our work practice? Aust N Z J Public Health 1999; 23(2):213–214.

38. Bin-Sallick M. Cultural safety: let's name it! Aust J Indigenous Educ 2003; 32:21–28.

39. Atkinson J. The healing power of educaring: capacity building through honouring and building cultural capital. Lismore, New South Wales: Submission to the Review of the Bachelor of Indigenous Studies, Southern Cross University; 2004.

40. Aboriginal peoples collection: mapping the healing journey. Final Report of a First National Research Project on Healing in Canadian Aboriginal Communities. Ottawa: Solicitor General Canada and the Aboriginal Healing Foundation; 2002.

Chapter 13

Gay and lesbian relationships and intimate partner abuse

Michael V Relf and Nancy Glass

Unfortunately, there aren't any shelters for men in the city. The only option I know of is a homeless shelter.

The response by a health care provider to a gay male seeking safety after his partner became physically abusive

CHAPTER CONTENTS

INTRODUCTION

Intimate partner abuse (IPA) battering, domestic violence, domestic abuse, spousal abuse, and intimate partner violence are all terms used to describe a similar phenomenon of violence and abuse in intimate relationships. However, associated with these terms are stereotypes and theoretical conceptualizations that men are the perpetrators and women victims, inherently implying that the phenomenon only occurs in opposite-sex intimate relationships.

The literature has identified a growing body of evidence about relationship development, conflict resolution, and IPA in same-sex relationships.[1-9] Despite this expanding body of knowledge, many clinicians, researchers, and law enforcement agencies, as well as IPA advocates and service agencies, are not aware of the scope of the problem and are ill-prepared to respond to, and treat the victims and perpetrators of same-sex IPA. Therefore, the purpose of this chapter is to provide a state-of-the-science critique about IPA in same-sex relationships while exploring the antecedents and outcomes associated with IPA in gay and lesbian relationships.

Throughout this chapter, the term *gay* is used to refer to a male who is in an intimate relationship with, or prefers, a same-sex partner, while the term *lesbian* refers to a female who is in an intimate relationship with, or prefers, a same-sex partner. In addition, men who have sex with men, or MSM, will also be utilized in this chapter to refer to men who engage in sex with other men, yet may not identify as gay. The word *partner* refers to a person of romantic interest or commitment partner.[1]

THEORETICAL PERSPECTIVES AND LESBIAN AND GAY IPA

With the evolving study of gay and lesbian IPA, theoretical controversy has evolved because 'if women batter, theories based on sexism and abuse of gender-based power' become insufficient to explain all forms of violence.[10] Using a gender-based orientation, batterers are labelled 'he' and victims 'she'. Consequently, lesbian and gay perpetrators and victims disappear.[11] Focusing on IPA within the confines of socially recognized marriage or relationships frequently results in the non-existence of same-sex IPA. Furthermore, codified laws that establish the legal parameters for defining IPA, ensuring services and providing protection for heterosexual persons, only further oppress the victims and perpetrators of same-sex IPA. As a result, the 'illegitimate' same-sex victims of IPA all too often find services to be scarce or non-existent.[11]

METHODOLOGICAL ISSUES IN RESEARCH

Several methodological challenges and issues limit the interpretation of findings from previous studies on gay and lesbian IPA. Prevalence estimates are often based on small samples or samples of convenience and subsequently do not represent the general population of gays and lesbians. Previous studies have used various definitions of abuse, time frames for measuring victimization and perpetration, and sampling procedures; therefore, findings are difficult to compare across studies and nations.[2,4] Despite the shortcomings and methodological challenges, findings from previous research provide an important context to understand the magnitude of the issue in which to develop future research studies and implement interventions.

Of the instruments frequently used to identify IPA, there is insensitivity to issues associated with same-sex IPA. For example, a powerful form of coercive control among gays and lesbians is the threat to 'out' the partner to family, an employer, or others. Additionally, the threat of unsafe sex or deliberate infection with HIV among gay men is also a powerful mechanism of control not explicated in any of the existing tools utilized in IPA screening and research. Table 13.1 provides one example of a screening tool for IPA that is relevant to gays and lesbians.

Obtaining accurate prevalence estimates

Accurately separating victim from perpetrator is necessary in order to estimate the prevalence of abuse victimization and perpetration in same-sex relationships.[12,13] The concept of 'mutual combat' is often assumed in same-sex relationships since both partners are of the same gender and equally capable of committing violence.[7] Although gay men and lesbians may use violence to defend themselves, frequently they question whether they were battered if they responded only once to the violence against them with violence of their own.[7] In a USA study of victimized lesbians, 78% reported attempts to defend themselves through physical force.[14]

In estimating prevalence of IPA in female same-sex relationships, researchers have not excluded IPA perpetrated by former male partners.[4] Thus, it is critical to delineate gender in order to gain a clearer picture of differences in IPA estimates between lesbian and heterosexual women.

Under-reporting of abuse in same-sex relationships

Similar to IPA in heterosexual relationships, abuse in same-sex relationships is under-reported. Because of societal homophobia, community denial, and lack of gay-sensitive and appropriate IPA resources, lesbian and gay victims of IPA frequently do not report IPA to the authorities, nor do they seek help. Many lesbians and gays perceive law enforcement agencies to be homophobic and heterosexist.[7]. Substantial evidence exists which illustrates the anti-gay violence allowed by law enforcement and committed by law enforcement agencies themselves. In a USA survey, 20% of anti-gay victimization was committed by the police in the form of physical and verbal abuse, entrapment, blackmail, and deliberate mishandling of anti-gay violence cases. Consequently, victims of same-sex IPA frequently do not report the abuse to police in order to avoid further verbal and physical abuse as well as discrimination.[15]

For abused lesbians and gays, there is often no place to turn for help and to escape the violence. Although lesbians can usually locate shelter services in the community, too often these shelters are not sensitive to the issues associated with same-sex IPA. In contrast, gay men seeking shelter from violence

Table 13.1 Same-Sex Battering Risk Assessment Tool[57]

SCREENING QUESTIONS
- In the past year, how many same-sex intimate partners have you had?
- Since coming 'out', how many same-sex intimate partners have you had?
- In the past five years, how many same-sex intimate partners have you had?

TIMEFRAME FOR ASSESSMENT
- During the *past year*, has a same-sex intimate partner . . .
- During the *past five years*, has a same-sex intimate partner
- Has a same-sex intimate partner *ever* . . .

1a. physically hurt you?
1b. threatened you?
2a. hit you with a hand or fist?
2b. slapped you?
2c. thrown something at you?
2d. pushed or shoved you?
2e. kicked you?
2f. hit you with an object?
3a. verbally threatened you?
3b. made fun of your appearance?
3c. verbally demeaned you?
3d. verbally demeaned you in front of others?
3e. forced you to get high?
3f. forced you to get drunk?
3g. intentionally 'outed' you to someone you did not want to know your sexual orientation?
4a. forced you to have sex when you didn't want to?
4b. refused to practice safe sex when you wanted to?
4c. forced you to do something sexually you didn't like to do?
4d. threatened to intentionally infect you with HIV?
5a. prevent you from leaving the house?
5b. getting a job?
5c. seeking or spending time with friends?
5d. continuing your education?
6a. intentionally destroyed things you care about?
6b. stolen your things?
6c. stalked you?
7a. made you feel like you were in danger?
7b. threatened you with a gun or weapon?
7c. made you feel afraid to go home?

often do not have safe places in the local community. Consequently, the magnitude of the problem continues to be under-reported.

Sampling lesbian and gay populations

One of the most difficult methodological challenges in the scientific study of gay and lesbian health and social issues is determining how to obtain a representative sample. Most studies have utilized samples obtained through gay and lesbian bars, social and support groups, and gay, lesbian, bisexual and transgender (GLBT) organizations. While these studies may accurately represent subsets of the gay and lesbian populations, they are not representative of the population in the larger communities.[1,4] Sampling for studies on IPA in the gay and lesbian community is further complicated by fear of exposure of same-sex relationships: potential participants are not publicly 'out' about their sexuality or they do not identify as gay or lesbian. Large representative surveys usually lack questions that would assist men and women to disclose their sexuality.

PREVALENCE OF IPA IN SAME-SEX RELATIONSHIPS

Prevalence estimates of IPA in same-sex relationships are based on limited samples because of some of the methodological challenges already outlined.

Male same-sex relationships

The only population-based study of IPA in male same-sex relationships using probability sampling techniques was in the USA.[16] Among this ethnically diverse sample of urban MSM (n = 2,881), the prevalence rates of IPA victimization were high. During the previous five years, 34% of urban MSM reported psychological abuse, 22.0% physical violence, and 5.1% sexual violence from a male partner or boyfriend. Eighteen per cent reported two or more types of IPA by a male intimate partner or boyfriend during the previous five years. Native American MSM reported the highest prevalence of all types of IPA except sexual abuse, where Latino MSM had the highest rate. In all categories of IPA, Asian/Pacific Islander MSM had the lowest prevalence rates of IPA victimization when compared with other racial/ethnic groups.

Female same-sex relationships

Several studies using convenience samples (i.e. women's festivals, lesbian organizations) have focused on IPA in lesbian relationships.[4,14,17–23] In these studies, between 17 and 52% of lesbians reported being abused by a current or former intimate partner. Importantly, most of the studies[4,14,18,20,21] clearly specified the gender of the perpetrator, but some did not.[24] It is very likely that some of the perpetrators were men from previous heterosexual relationships.[2]

In a survey comparing lesbian and heterosexual women drawn from the USA, physical abuse by a male partner in a committed relationship was reported by 27% of the heterosexual women.[18] Similarly, 25% of the lesbians in a committed relationship reported physical abuse.

In the large National Violence Against Women Survey conducted in the USA, 11.4% of the 79 women who had a history of living with a same-sex partner reported being physically and/or sexually abused by a female partner. Findings from these studies indicate that the prevalence of IPA in lesbian relationships is similar to the prevalence of IPA in heterosexual relationships.[2] Even at the lowest prevalence estimate reported (11%), IPA in lesbian relationships is a significant women's health and public health issue that is often ignored.

RISK FACTORS FOR IPA IN SAME-SEX RELATIONSHIPS

Although the evidence examining risk factors for IPA is limited, studies have consistently reported younger age, less education, prior childhood and adult physical and sexual violence, depression, HIV status, and alcohol and drug abuse as being associated with IPA in same-sex relationships. The following section reviews the risk factor evidence to assist clinicians in developing appropriate screening and intervention protocols for IPA.

Individual factors

Among urban MSM in the USA, age and education were associated with all forms of IPA.[16] Younger MSM (under 40 years) were more likely than older MSM (60 years or older) to experience sexual IPA. MSM with graduate or professional degrees were less likely to experience any form of IPA compared to MSM with less education. Physical and psychological abuse were more likely to be found among HIV-positive men, and less likely to be found among MSM who have never tested for HIV.

Among lesbians, study participants are remarkably similar in terms of demographics. The majority of lesbian participants across the research literature on female same-sex IPA are young (20–40 years of age), middle class, college-educated, Caucasian women. This probably reflects the sampling methods, which are limited in terms of demographic representation, and must be interpreted with caution.[1]

Childhood and adult exposure to violence

Several studies have examined the association between childhood victimization and subsequent involvement in an abusive relationship among lesbians[13,14,19,20,22,25–27] and gay men.[2,25,26,28–32] Lesbians who experienced victimization in the home as children were more likely to be abused in their intimate relationships as adults, to be abusive in their relationships, or both, when compared with lesbians who did not experience abuse as children.[13,20] In a small study of lesbians ($n = 40$), 73% reported witnessing parental aggression or experienced aggression in their family of origin.[14]

Among Latino gay men in the USA, experiencing childhood sexual abuse increased the likelihood for IPA in adulthood.[33] Similarly, Relf and colleagues[34] demonstrated that urban MSM in the USA who experienced childhood sexual abuse were more likely to be battered by a boyfriend or male intimate partner in adulthood.

Other studies have found contradictory findings related to the association of childhood victimization and adult exposure to IPA.[25,26] The studies on the role of childhood victimization and exposure to adult IPA are limited because the majority use small, non-random samples and none of the studies included heterosexual women or men. Therefore a comparison of rates of childhood victimization between gay and lesbian and heterosexual men and women is not possible.[2,4]

Abuse in a past adult relationship, especially a heterosexual relationship, was associated with abuse in current lesbian relationships either as a victim, perpetrator, or both.[20]

Substance use

Correlation studies have demonstrated the relationship between substance use and IPA in female same-sex relationships.[12,14,15,19] In a small survey study (n = 104) drawn from the USA,[12] frequency of alcohol use was associated with the number and types of abusive acts both perpetrated and experienced from an intimate partner, but drug use was not correlated with abusive behaviour. Renzetti[14,17] found that general use of substances by either or both partners was correlated with abusive actions. When examining differences between violent and non-violent lesbian relationships, Lie and colleagues identified that substance use was generally present in the violent lesbian relationships;[19] however, the study did not examine the use of substances by partners during the actual incidents of IPA.

Among gay men, substance use has been demonstrated to increase risk for IPA.[33–38] In a qualitative study of 25 gay men from the USA in which IPA was present in the relationship, 13 of the respondents identified alcohol as a precipitating factor to IPA while 3 believed that alcohol or drugs were used as a result of IPA.[37] When examining the relationship between substance use and IPA among MSM, Relf and colleagues[34] demonstrated that heavy drinking, problems with alcohol use, number of drugs used, and sex with a male while under the influence of alcohol or drugs was causally related to IPA among urban MSM. Similarly, Stermac and colleagues studied 29 males who reported to a sexual assault crisis unit at a university teaching hospital in Toronto, Canada during a 15 month period. In this study 86% of the sexual assaults were perpetrated by another male and victims of the sexual assault frequently reported use of alcohol (46%) and drugs (18%) prior to the assault.

Among Latin-American MSM (n = 273) from New York City who were the victims of IPA, 50% stated that they were sometimes or always under the influence of alcohol and/or drugs when the battering occurred.[33] In this study, use of marijuana and cocaine/crack were strongly associated with being a victim of abuse.

Depression

Clinicians must be alert to the signs and symptoms of depression in lesbians and gays with a history of IPA. Victimization as an adult by an intimate partner has been positively correlated with depression in both lesbians and gays.[39] Low self-esteem was found to be the strongest predictor of depression among a large sample of lesbians and gays.[39] Among urban MSMs, Relf and colleagues demonstrated that aversive emotions – depression, well-being, and suicidality – were causally associated with IPA. Among MSMs who have experienced non-consensual sex with another male in adulthood, there was an increased probability of ever being diagnosed with a mood disorder, being currently depressed, and experiencing suicidal ideation.[38]

Controlling and dependent behaviour

Desire for control over resources and decision-making in relationships has no sexual orientation boundaries.[40] Investigators have examined the role of controlling and jealous behaviour, dependency, and power in abusive same-sex female relationships.[13,4,7,19] In contrast, however, no research was identified examining this phenomenon among gay men.

Among lesbian couples who reported a need to share all family and social activities, IPA was more likely to be part of the relationship.[13] Renzetti[14,17] found that abusive lesbians were more dependent on their intimate partner. Furthermore, the study reported that the greater the respondent's desire to be independent and the greater the abusive partner's dependency, the more likely the abusive partner was to inflict numerous types of abuse with greater frequency.

BARRIERS TO DISCLOSURE OF IPA

Several individual and societal factors have been examined as potential barriers to disclosure of same-sex IPA to health professionals, criminal justice, law enforcement, or advocates. These barriers include internalized homophobia; fear of disclosure of sexual orientation to family, friends, employer, co-workers; societal homophobia; and lack of existing health and social services in the community.

Internalized homophobia

Internalized homophobia has been defined as the internalization by sexual minorities of negative attitudes and assumptions about homosexuality.[41,42] It has been associated with lower social support, lack of connection to community, loneliness, low self-esteem, and depression.[41] Sexual minorities in abusive relationships may deny or doubt her/his sexuality, feeling that the IPA was caused by their sexual orientation.[43] This internalized homophobia or denying of sexual orientation may prevent victims and perpetrators from seeking help for IPA and increase the risk of repeat abuse. Among gay men, internalized homophobia has been linked to IPA.[44]

Fear of disclosure

Some victims of same-sex IPA, like heterosexual victims, have difficulty identifying their experiences as abusive. As indicated in several studies,[45–47] individuals in same-sex relationships may be at additional risk from the fear of disclosing their homosexual relationship to family, friends, employers, neighbours, health care professionals, or law enforcement officers. This is related to the stigma attached by society and a lack of community and advocacy services specific to same-sex relationships.

Due to gender role expectations, as well as societal expectations of males, gay men who are the victims of IPA may have even greater difficulty disclosing the abuse and victimization. Although there has been growing awareness of the IPA problem as a result of the domestic violence movement, there has been virtual silence about same-sex IPA.[7] Consequently, many gay men may have never heard of gay domestic violence. Often gay men are not able to see themselves as victims simply because of their male gender.[7] Furthermore, individuals who live in areas with a small gay and lesbian community fear that the community may discover what happened. The victim or perpetrator may be a prominent, well-liked, and outspoken advocate in the community, thus making seeking assistance from within the community difficult, for fear of losing friends and support systems, as well as shame.

Societal homophobia

Homophobia, the irrational fear, hatred, and intolerance of homosexuality, and heterosexism operate so that physical and sexual abuse in same-sex relationships is ignored or not taken seriously by the health care and criminal justice systems. Homophobia and heterosexism does not cause IPA in same-sex relationships: however, it does create an opportune environment that supports the abusive behavior.[17,41,43,45,48] Homophobia creates isolation and invisibility and may contribute to the risk of IPA. Victims are given the message that the abuse is tolerated by the lack of health care, criminal justice, and community resources that fail to target individuals in same-sex relationships. Perpetrators clearly get the message that there will not be negative consequences for abusing their partner 'in that kind of relationship'.[45]

To admit that physical and sexual abuse occurs in same-sex intimate relationships means to accept that individuals engage in intimate sexual relationships with others of the same sex. Despite the fact that IPA is about power and control, to examine female perpetrators and female victims or male perpetrators and male victims requires society to think about same-sex relationships. This is a mental image that many in our society, including some of those in the health care system, are not prepared to face.[17,41,43,45,48–50]

LIMITED EXISTING SERVICES AND TRAINING

Although a number of domestic violence agencies and community organizations have worked to raise awareness of IPA in same-sex relationships, many obstacles to adequately addressing IPA in this population remain.[1,2,4] Studies have demonstrated that victims of same-sex IPA turn most often to friends or mental health providers for support[17,48–50] rather than accessing resources through community agencies. For example, women in same-sex relationships report not utilizing domestic violence agency services such as hotlines, support groups, or legal advocacy because of the perception that services are targeted at heterosexual women abused by men.[17,43]

When domestic violence agencies do targeted outreach, make a commitment to staff education and training, and provide programmes such as sexual minority support groups with trained staff, victims and perpetrators utilize the services.

HEALTH OUTCOMES OF IPA IN SAME–SEX RELATIONSHIPS

The consequences of gay and lesbian victimization range from the short-term and relatively 'minor behavioral and psychological reactions such as headaches, increased agitation and sleep disturbances to long-term and more severe reactions such as depression, increased drug use, uncontrollable crying and post-traumatic stress disorder.'[39]

Among heterosexual women, forced sex by a male partner increased the rate of pelvic inflammatory disease, increased the risk of sexually transmitted diseases (STDs), and was associated with unexplained vaginal bleeding and other genitourinary-related health problems.[51,52] However, no literature was identified demonstrating the physiological outcomes of IPA in lesbian relationships. Two studies have indicated that rape[2] and unwanted penetration[4] were common in gay men. Therefore, it is reasonable to assume that forced sex among MSM increases the risk of HIV and other STDs and may be associated with colorectal-related health problems, if anal intercourse was involved.

Examining battering as a factor associated with HIV-risky behaviour, Merrill and Wolfe[53] identified that 13% ($n = 7$) of the battered gay/bisexual men seeking services for IPA ($n = 52$) reported that the perpetrating partner sometimes or frequently tried to infect, or infected them with HIV. Three of these men (5.7%) reported HIV seroconversion as a consequence of IPA from their HIV-positive male partner. Similarly, among a convenience sample of 307 Latin American MSM in New York City, men who engaged in unprotected receptive anal sex with a male lover were more likely to be physically and sexually abused by any partner.[33]

Exploring the relationship of physical violence and a diagnosis of HIV, Greenwood and colleagues[16] identified that HIV-positive MSMs are 1.5 times more likely to be physically battered by a male intimate partner than HIV-negative persons. Supporting this finding, Relf and colleagues identified that IPA is causally related to HIV-risk behaviours among a probability-based sample of urban MSMs.[34] Furthermore, in a nationally representative probability sample of HIV-positive adult patients in primary care in the USA ($n = 2,864$),[44] 11.5% of the MSMs had experienced physical violence by a partner or other important person since HIV diagnosis; 4.5% of this sample related the physical violence to their HIV status.

The most severe outcome of IPA is homicide. In a surveillance report for homicide among intimate partners in the US between 1981 and 1998,[54] investigators identified that the proportion of intimate partner homicide (IPH) committed by same-sex partners was greater for gay men than lesbians. Among the male victims, a large percentage of the total IPH was by a boyfriend (32.5%) or same-sex partner (6.2%). Similarly, among female victims, a large percentage was by a girlfriend (34.7%) or same-sex partner (0.5%).

Glass and colleagues[55] conducted a case study to examine female-perpetrated intimate partner femicide ($n = 5$) and attempted femicide in same-sex relationships ($n = 4$). Among the nine cases, prior physical violence, controlling behaviours, jealousy, alcohol and drugs, and ending the relationship were consistently reported antecedents to the incident. These findings, although preliminary, indicate that power and control are central to models of IP femicide and attempted femicide, whether perpetrated by a man or a woman.

IMPLICATIONS FOR CLINICAL PRACTICE

In addressing IPA in gay and lesbian intimate relationships, numerous obstacles must be overcome. First, nearly all health professionals lack awareness that this problem exists.[53] Just as in opposite-sex relationships, physical, psychological, emotional, and sexual abuse do not constitute normal partner dynamics in same-sex couples.[16]

Assessing for IPA in gay and lesbian relationships

Through asking about IPA in all relationships, a critical opportunity to facilitate disclosure of IPA victimization is offered. Additionally, it facilitates the health provider's ability to develop a plan to protect safety and improve the client's health and well-being.[56] Providing health care services to gays and lesbians is often complicated by provider insensitivity, bias, homophobia, lack of understanding, and lack of training.[57]

'Multiple screenings by skilled health providers, when conducted face-to-face, markedly increase the identification of domestic violence.'[56] Therefore, asking, as opposed to indicator-based screening, grants the clinician an increased opportunity to identify and intervene when symptoms are the result of IPA. When assessing gays and lesbians for IPA, the use of non-biased terminology is critical. By minimizing the use of the heterosexual viewpoint (husband, wife) and using terms such as partner, the battered victim is afforded an opportunity to respond without simultaneously having to disclose his or her homosexuality.[57] Table 13.1 provides a guide to assessment questions that can be used for assessing IPA in same-sex couples.

Assessing for, and responding to IPA in same-sex couples requires that all responders (e.g. police, paramedics) and health care providers (e.g. physicians, nurses, social workers, psychologists) are not only alert to signs of IPA but also sensitive to issues surrounding homosexuality.[53] This includes not only assessing for physical abuse but also emotional abuse, sexual abuse, financial abuse, and intimidation, coercion, control, and isolation.[57]

Members of the health care team should suspect IPA when acute physical manifestations such as contusions, lacerations, fractures, abdominal trauma, head trauma, or oropharyngeal/vaginal/anal trauma exist. Similarly, with chronic health conditions, including pain syndromes and gastrointestinal disorders, health professionals should ask carefully about IPA.[57-59] Clinicians must also be aware of the less obvious signs and symptoms. In some same-sex relationships, STDs, including HIV, may indicate sexual risk-taking or relationship difficulties, requiring further exploration and referral, as appropriate.[57] Additionally, the destructive consequences of IPA can be exhibited by depression, suicidal ideation/suicide attempts, post-traumatic stress disorder, alcoholism, and substance use.[58] Therefore, health professionals working with same-sex couples must be cognizant of the multiple types of IPA utilized and thoroughly evaluate the origin of the physical, sexual, emotional, or psychological injury or symptoms identified during examination.[58]

IMPLICATIONS FOR RESEARCH AND POLICY

To gain a more comprehensive understanding of same-sex IPA, theory-driven, well-controlled, mixed-methodological studies are needed.[16,53,60] To expand the current knowledge of same-sex IPA, gays and lesbians in middle-sized urban, small cities and rural communities as well as urban settings must be included. Similarly, sampling strategies must include a range of ages, racial and ethnic minorities, and non-gay identified individuals in same-sex intimate relationships. Future research must also examine sex-role attitudes related to aggression since it is presumed that they are different, based on gender and sexual orientation. Finally, research examining same-sex IPA needs to include lesbian, gay, and heterosexual comparison samples so that the current knowledge of same-sex IPA can be clarified and expanded.

Almost no literature currently exists about the perpetrators of same-sex IPA. Without assessing both sides of IPA in same-sex relationships, interventions and community responses will be ineffective and incomplete. Furthermore, intervention research, both at the intimate partner dyad level and the community level, is required. Moreover, longitudinal, cost-effectiveness, and best-practices research is essential to determine effectiveness of prevention, screening, and treatment interventions for same-sex victims and perpetrators of IPA.

As gay and lesbian victims of IPA have not been granted equal treatment under the legal system, social analysis and interventions aimed at influencing policy and legislative change are crucial.[61] At the local level, community domestic violence experts, as well as victims, can work for policy and procedural reform. The first step to achieve this outcome is to conduct community surveys to determine the incidence of IPA victimization and perpetration in the gay and lesbian community. Equally important, surveys are also needed to assess victims' experiences with police, the courts, and other protective and social service agencies.[61]

Empowered by data, advocates can develop training programmes for the police and legal system as well as seek funding for community service agencies that are gay and lesbian sensitive and accessible. Finally, social analyses and evaluation research, such as a court-watch programme to monitor prosecution and sentencing patterns in cases involving same-sex IPA, aimed at impacting policy and legislative change, are crucial.[61]

CONCLUSION

IPA among gay and lesbian persons is a serious public health issue. Victimization rates appear to equal or exceed the rates of women in heterosexual relationships. As in opposite-sex relationships, correlates of IPA victimization and perpetration are multifaceted. However, because of the lack of clinician recognition, and internalized and societal homophobia, as well as clinician lack of sensitivity and training, this detrimental phenomenon is not assessed for in the health care setting. Future research is needed to critically examine this phenomenon using mixed methods, longitudinal, well-controlled studies that are representative of all gays and lesbians. Additionally, societal and structural interventions are needed to increase recognition, and to facilitate availability of resources for both victims and perpetrators, as well as to eliminate the stigma and prejudice associated with same-sex IPA.

ACKNOWLEDGEMENTS

The authors would like to thank Anna Ford, student at the Georgetown University School of Nursing and Health Studies, Washington, DC, for her assistance in collecting the literature reviewed in this chapter.

REFERENCES

1. Burke LK, Follingstad DR. Violence in lesbian and gay relationships: theory, prevalence and correlational factors. Clin Psych Rev 1999; 19(5):487–512.
2. Tjaden P, Thoennes N, Allison CJ. Comparing violence over the lifespan in samples of same-sex and opposite sex cohabitants. Violence Vict 1999; 14:413–425.
3. Merrill G. Understanding domestic violence among gay and bisexual men. In: Berger RK, ed. Issues in domestic violence. Thousand Oaks, CA: Sage; 1998.
4. Waldner-Haugrud LK, Vaden Gratch L. Sexual coercion in gay/lesbian relationships: descriptive and gender differences. Violence Vict 1997; 12:87–98.
5. Waldner-Haugrud LK, Vaden Gratch L, Magruder B. Victimization and perpetration rates of violence in gay and lesbian relationships: gender issues explored. Violence Vict 1997; 12(2):173–184.
6. Kurdek LA. Conflict resolution styles in gay, lesbian, heterosexual non-parent and heterosexual parent couples. J Marriage Fam 1994; 6(3):705–722.
7. Letellier P. Gay and bisexual male domestic violence victimization: challenges to feminist theory and responses to violence. Violence Vict 1994; 9(2):95–106.
8. Berger RM. Men together: understanding the gay couple. J Homosex 1990; 19(3):31–49.
9. Campbell JC, Humphreys J. Nursing care of survivors of family violence. St. Louis: Mosby;1993.
10. Hamberger LK. Domestic partner abuse: expanding paradigms for understanding and intervention. Violence Vict 1994; 9(2):91–94.
11. Bograd M. Strengthening domestic violence theories: intersection of race, class, sexual orientation, and gender. J Marital Fam Ther 1999; 25(3):275–289.
12. Schilit R, Lie G, Montagne, M. Substance use as a correlate of violence in intimate lesbian relationships. J Homosex 1990; 19:51–65.
13. Lockhart L, White BA, Causby V, et al. Letting out the secret: violence in lesbian relationships. J Interpers Violence 1994; 9(4):469–493.
14. Renzetti CM. Violence in lesbian relationships: a preliminary analysis of causal factors. J Interpers Violence 1998; 3(4):7–27.
15. Herek GM. The context of anti-gay violence: notes on cultural and psychological heterosexism. J Interpers Violence 1990; 5:315–333.
16. Greenwood G, Relf M, Huang B, et al. Battering victimization among a probability-based sample of men who have sex with men (MSM). Am J Public Health 2002; 92(12):1964–1969.
17. Renzetti CM. Violent betrayal: partner abuse in lesbian relationships. Newbury Park, CA: Sage; 1992.
18. Brand P, Kidd A. Frequency of physical aggression in heterosexual and female homosexual dyads. Psych Rep 1986; 5:1307–1313.
19. Coleman VE. Lesbian battering: the relationship between personality and the perpetration of violence. Violence Vict 1994; 9(2):139–152.
20. Lie GW, Schilit R, Bush J, et al. Lesbian in currently aggressive relationships: how frequently do they report aggressive past relationships. Violence Vict 1991; 6:121–135.
21. Lie GW, Gentlewarrior S. Intimate violence in lesbian relationships: discussion of survey findings and practice implications. J Soc Serv Res 1991; 15:41–59.
22. Loulan J. Lesbian passion: loving ourselves and each other. San Francisco: Spinsters/Aunt Late; 1987.
23. Schilit R, Lie G, Montagne M. Substance use as a correlate of violence in intimate lesbian relationships. J Homosex 1990; 19:51–65.
24. Waterman CK, Dawson LJ, Bologna MJ. Sexual coercion in gay male and lesbian relationships: predictors and implications for support services. J Sex Res 1989; 26:118–124.

25. Coleman VE. Violence between lesbian couples: a between groups comparison. Unpublished doctoral dissertation. (University Microfilms International, 9109022): 1991.

26. Kelly EE, Warshafsy L. Partner abuse in gay male and lesbian couples. Paper presented at the Third National Conference for Family Violence Researchers. Durham, NH; 1987.

27. Bradford J, Ryan C, Rothblum ED. National lesbian health care survey: implications for mental health care. J Consult Clin Psychol 1994; 62(2):228–242.

28. Duncan DF. Prevalence of sexual assault victimization among heterosexual and gay/lesbian university students. Psychol Bull 1990; 66:65–66.

29. Doll L, Bartholow B, Joy D, et al. Self-reported childhood and adolescent sexual abuse among adult homosexual and bisexual men. Child Abuse Neglect 1992; 16:855–864.

30. Paul J, Catania J, Pollack L, et al. Understanding childhood sexual abuse as a predictor of sexual risk-taking among men who have sex with men: the Urban Men's Health Study. Child Abuse Neglect 2001; 25(4):557–584.

31. Lenderking WR, Wold C, Mayer KH, et al. Childhood sexual abuse among homosexual men: prevalence and association with unsafe sex. J Gen Intern Med 1997; 12(4):250–253.

32. Jinich S, Paul JP, Stall R, et al. Childhood sexual abuse and HIV risk-taking behavior among gay and bisexual men. AIDS Behav 1998; 2(1):41–51.

33. Nieves-Rosa LE, Carballo-Dieguez A, Dolezal C. Domestic abuse and HIV-risk behavior in Latin American men who have sex with men in New York City. J Gay Lesbian Soc Serv 2000; 11(1):77–90.

34. Relf MV, Huang B, Campbell J, et al. Gay identity, interpersonal violence, and HIV risk behaviors: empirically testing theoretical relationships among a probability based sample of urban MSM. J Assoc Nurses AIDS Care 2004; 15(2):14–26.

35. Zierler S, Cunningham WE, Anderson R, et al. Violence victimization after HIV infection in a probability sample of adult patients in primary care. Am J Public Health 2000; 90(2):208–215.

36. Stermac L, Sheridan PM, Davidson A, et al. Sexual assault of adult males. J Interpers Violence 1996; 11(1):52–64.

37. Cruz JM, Peralta RL. Family violence and substance use: the perceived effects of substance use within gay male relationships. Violence Vict 2001; 16(2):161–172.

38. Ratner PA, Johnson JL, Shoveller JA, et al. Non-consensual sex experienced by men who have sex with men: prevalence and association with mental health. Patient Educ Couns 2003; 49(1):67–74.

39. Otis MD, Skinner WF. The prevalence of victimization and its effect on mental well-being among lesbian and gay people. J Homosex 1996; 30(3):93–121.

40. Miller SL. Expanding the boundaries: toward a more inclusive and integrated study of intimate violence. Violence Vict 1994; 9(2):183–194.

41. Balsam KF. Nowhere to hide: lesbian IPA, homophobia and minority stress. In: Kaschak E, ed. Intimate betrayal: domestic violence in lesbian relationships. New York: Haworth Press; 2001.

42. Sophie J. Internalized homophobia and lesbian identity. J Homosex 1987; 14:53–65.

43. Girshick L. No sugar, no spice: reflections on research on women-to-women sexual violence. Violence Against Women 2002; 8(12):1500–1520.

44. Zierler S, Cunningham WE, Anderson R, et al. Violence victimization after HIV infection in a probability sample of adult patients in primary care. Am J Public Health 2000; 90(2):208–215.

45. Worcester N. Women's use of force: complexities and challenges of taking the issue seriously. Violence Against Women 2002; 8(11):1390–1413.

46. Kuenle K, Sullivan A. Gay and lesbian victimization: reporting factors in domestic violence and bias incidents. Crim Justice Behav 2003; 30(1):85–96.

47. Duffy A, Momirov J. Family violence: a Canadian introduction. Toronto: James Lorimer; 1997.

48. Giorgio G. Speaking silence: definitional dialogues in abusive lesbian relationships. Violence Against Women 2002; 8(1):1233–1259.

49. Ristock JL. Understanding violence in lesbian relationships: an examination of misogyny and homophobia. Can Womens Stud 1991; 12:74–79.

50. Ristock JL. No more secrets: violence in lesbian relationship. New York: Routledge; 2002.
51. Campbell JC, Soeken KL. Women's responses to battering: a test of a model. Res Nurs Health 1999; 22(1):49–58.
52. Campbell JC, Woods AB, Chouaf KL, et al. Reproductive health consequences of intimate partner violence: a nursing research review. Clin Nurs Res 2000; 9(3):217–237.
53. Merrill GS, Wolfe VA. Battered gay men: an exploration of abuse, help-seeking, and why they stay. J Homosex 2000; 39(2):1–30.
54. Paulozzi LJ, Saltzman LE, Thompson MP, et al. Surveillance for homicide among intimate partners: United States, 1981–1998. MMWR CDC Surveill Summ 2001; 50(SS03):1–16.
55. Glass NE, Koziol-McLain J, Campbell JC, et al. Female perpetrated femicide and attempted femicide: a case study. Violence Against Women. In Press.
56. The Family Violence Prevention Fund. Preventing domestic violence: clinical guidelines on routine screening. San Francisco: The Family Violence Prevention Fund; 1999.
57. Relf MV. Battering and HIV in men who have sex with men: a critique and synthesis of the literature. J Assoc Nurses AIDS Care 200112(3):17–24.
58. Eyler AE, Cohen M. Case studies in partner violence. Am Fam Physician 1999; 60(9):2569–2576.
59. Campbell JC, Lewendowski L. Mental and physical health effects of intimate partner violence on women and children. Psych Clin N Am 1997; 20(2):353–374.
60. Burke LK, Follingstad DR. Violence in lesbian and gay relationships: theory, prevalence and correlational factors. Clin Psych Rev 1999; 19(5):487–512.
61. Hamberger LK. Domestic partner abuse: expanding paradigms for understanding and intervention. Violence Vict 1994; 9(2):91–94.

Chapter 14

Intimate partner abuse research and training: the way forward

Kelsey Hegarty, Gene Feder, and Gwenneth Roberts

This book has demonstrated that for such a common problem in health settings (Chapter 2), with significant morbidity and mortality (Chapter 3), the current literature (Chapters 5 and 6) has little robust evidence to inform the identification and management of intimate partner abuse (IPA). Similarly, although researchers have not systematically studied the effects of social and cultural victimization, authors in a number of chapters have described the importance of understanding how gender, ethnicity, sexual orientation, disability, and socioeconomic status affect an individual's experience of abuse. A powerful source of evidence is women's stories of their paths through violence and abuse (Chapter 12) and these can inform health professionals how best to assist them in their journeys.

This book has not addressed primary prevention – reducing the societal prevalence of abuse. However, health professionals who reinforce the unacceptability of IPA in the community may contribute to the political and cultural challenge to abuse that is part of primary prevention. We need to understand the individual and social power dynamics that produce and maintain abuse and affect its impact on women. Using a broad framework, abuse must be viewed in terms of gender, recognizing progress towards gender equality as an essential component of primary prevention at one level. The authors are aware that intervention for IPA involves more than the health sector, and there are many parts of this book where inter-sectoral and multi-agency collaboration is reinforced.

Recommendations for training and research in the future conclude this book. Future research and training need to take into account not only the limitations of knowledge about IPA but also the biases and prejudices of health professionals, which reflect societal attitudes.

WHAT DO WE KNOW ABOUT IPA?

Chapter 1 demonstrated that IPA is an ancient and often hidden problem. It is only in the last 30 years that IPA has taken its place on the public agenda and therefore presented a challenge to health professionals. During that time research has revealed that women who have experienced IPA attend health services frequently. The significant impact of IPA on women's physical and mental health is well documented in Chapter 3. More recent research, described in Chapter 8, has measured the detrimental effects on children who live in families where violence and abuse take place. We know that the likelihood of experiencing intimate partner abuse as an adult is high if you are a woman and have witnessed abuse at home during your childhood.

Qualitative research, described in Chapter 5, tells us that women want health professionals to listen to and believe them, be non-judgemental, and support them in their decisions. We know that some health professionals fail to inquire about IPA and for some women there are negative outcomes upon disclosure. Although health professionals subscribe to the ethical practice of 'do no harm', because of lack of training and knowledge some women are further victimized in health care systems. Furthermore, women tell us that there is a lack of response from others such as police and the legal professionals.

Most of the early research has focused on women as victims; later research has investigated particular groups such as women in their childbearing years (Chapter 7), non-English-speaking women in Western countries (Chapter 11), Indigenous women (Chapter 12), and women with disabilities (Chapter 9). Other areas remain where research is in its infancy, such as perpetrators (Chapter 9), and abuse between same-sex couples (Chapter 13). We know that health professionals have to rethink the concept that IPA occurs only in opposite-sex relationships as they are often ill-prepared to respond to, and treat, the victims and perpetrators of same-sex IPA.

WHAT DON'T WE KNOW ABOUT IPA?

Many conundrums remain about what is the best way to help women who are experiencing or have experienced partner abuse. Controversy surrounds issues such as screening in health care settings (Chapter 5), and the mandatory reporting of IPA (Chapter 10). Current research is investigating whether women will benefit from a variety of interventions such as screening, advocacy, counselling, and referral in health care settings (Chapter 6). It is likely to be that no single intervention will benefit all women. We know even less about what works for women of different cultural and ethnic backgrounds, for Indigenous peoples, and for same-sex couples.

TRAINING AND EDUCATION

Chapter 4 gives a comprehensive overview of education and training for health professionals about how to address IPA. It suggests that there needs to be mainstreaming of training in undergraduate and postgraduate teaching of health professionals. Currently this training is marginal or completely absent. Participation in training is frequently voluntary so that sessions are often 'preaching to the converted'. Existing programmes have had limited evaluation and insufficient attention is given to the organizational change that needs to occur for educational interventions to work.

Training programmes for health professionals need to incorporate knowledge of how common domestic violence is in general practice, emergency rooms, and mental health services. It is important for participants to understand the different types of abuse experienced by women, for example physical, sexual, emotional, and the consequences on women's emotional and physical well-being. Education programmes also need to address management strategies, not only for individual victim/survivors, but in how to manage the whole family, as described in Chapter 9. There are several ethical issues that need to be incorporated into IPA training. For example, it is inappropriate that women who are experiencing partner abuse and who are afraid of retribution from their partners, if the disclosure to the health professional is discovered, are referred for joint counselling. Such strategies are appropriate for marital conflict but not partner abuse because of the coercion and risk to safety that exist in intimate abusive relationships. Generally, the issue of confidentiality is central to an ethical response to domestic violence by health professionals it needs to be addressed in guidelines or training programmes on domestic violence.

In previous evaluations of continuing education, it has been constantly emphasized that the best methods of educating health professionals are those which are adult-learning focused, interactive, and targeted to the perceived needs of the participants, rather than didactic learning alone.[1] Methods used should include:

- consumer consultants;
- simulated patients;
- case discussions and peer support groups.

Evaluations of both undergraduate and continuing professional development of health professionals in the area of domestic violence have demonstrated the effective impact of patients presenting their own experiences, to allow interaction and further questioning from health professionals (Chapter 4). Standardized, or simulated patients (SPs) are persons (usually actors) trained to portray a patient with a particular presentation and can be used for teaching sensitive communication skills and for formative and summative evaluation.

IPA poses particular challenges to health professionals in the area of communication skills because of the sensitive nature of the problem. Training in this area should be increased in medical, nursing, and other health professional schools, postgraduate training programmes, and at a continuing professional development level. Only by changing education programmes and policies of institutions can alterations be made that might help women who experience IPA.

FUTURE RESEARCH DIRECTIONS

We work in an era of evidence-based health care, with a growing emphasis on using research findings to justify policy and clinical practice decisions. One of the most dramatic changes in the past 20 years in the discourse around health care is the focus on randomized controlled trial research evidence. The focus is explicitly on the efficacy and effectiveness of interventions, with the goal of basing policy and clinical practice decisions on patient-centred outcomes, like mortality, morbidity, and quality of life. The requirement for randomized controlled trial evidence is based on a particular view of methodological quality: 'the extent to which all aspects of a study's design and conduct can be shown to protect against systematic bias, non-systematic bias and inferential error.'[2] This definition underpins a hierarchy, with meta-analyses and randomized controlled trials at the top and observational studies and case reports at the bottom. Table 14.1 shows such a hierarchy.[3]

Application of this hierarchy to public health interventions[4] and broader health policy[5] is problematic. The exclusion of qualitative research reflects a judgement, not shared by qualitative researchers and many health professionals,[6] about the limited value of qualitative studies as a source of evidence about effectiveness. In the context of health care policy towards domestic violence, there are specific reasons why randomized controlled trials are not a secure basis for judging interventions.

Table 14.1 Evidence hierarchy for clinical guidance

Grade of recommendation	Level of evidence	Therapeutic or preventive interventions
A	1a	Systematic review of randomized controlled trials
	1b	Individual randomized controlled trial
	1c	All or none (met when *all* patients died before the treatment became available, but some now survive on it; or when some patients died before the treatment became available, but none now die on it)
B	2a	Systematic review of cohort studies
	2b	Individual cohort study (including low-quality randomized controlled trial e.g. <80% follow-up)
	2c	'Outcomes' research
	3a	Systematic review of case-control studies
	3b	Individual case-control study
C	4	Case-series (and poor-quality cohort and case-control studies)
D	5	Expert opinion without explicit critical appraisal, or based on physiology, bench research, or 'first principles'

First, randomization of women experiencing abuse to intervention and 'normal care' arms is logistically difficult and ethically questionable. Randomization by health care setting, such as general practices, antenatal clinics, or accident and emergency departments is more feasible, but the increased sample size of a cluster-randomized design creates an additional barrier to running such a trial. Second, the short time-scales of most trials mean that they are likely to miss potentially positive outcomes of domestic violence screening programmes where there is likely to be a long gap between the intervention and any measurable effect on participants' well-being. Third, there is still debate on appropriate outcome measures; different participants may have different goals in seeking help from the health care system and these will not necessarily be captured with standardized measures. Fourth, implementation of a domestic violence screening programme with a system of referral and follow-up is a complex intervention that will require tailoring to specific settings and may be difficult to standardize sufficiently to allow evaluation with a controlled trial design. There will remain a need for non-experimental quantitative studies that evaluate health service-based programmes for partner abuse, even if randomized controlled trials prove feasible and receive funding.

In addition to a wider range of quantitative study designs, we believe there is a central role for qualitative research in articulating what survivors of partner abuse want (or would have wanted) from health care professionals. When new interventions are implemented, we need studies exploring their feasibility and acceptability in addition to their overall effect on outcomes for women experiencing partner abuse.

We realize that even when we broaden the evidence base beyond controlled studies we are still limited by a framework that conceptualizes interventions in line with a medical model, albeit not a strictly biomedical one. Carole Warshaw and colleagues' (Chapter 4) critique of the strait jacket of the medical model on clinician's response to domestic violence is relevant here, and also discussed by Michael Rodriguez and George Saba in their exploration of cross-cultural competence (Chapter 11). Nevertheless we believe there is a role for conventional health services research in this field. A political case for this type of research is that it is the chief evidence currency for health policy makers and health service funders, and may help secure resources for domestic violence work in health care settings. We believe there is also a strong scientific case for applying quantitative research methods to single interventions and multi-faceted programmes to improve the response of clinical services to IPA. It is impossible to make evidence-based recommendations without rigorously testing interventions, taking into account potential harm as well as benefit of new programmes.

The evidence base supporting clinicians' choice of effective interventions for women experiencing partner abuse is small: the total number of primary studies covered by the reviews in Chapter 6 is 16, excluding those focusing on perpetrators. The studies mostly have weak study designs or are poorly reported, and most do not measure woman-centred outcomes. Yet, they do point to types of intervention that hold promise, in particular domestic violence advocacy and some psychological interventions.

Several methodological recommendations for future prevalence research are discussed in Chapter 2. It is important to measure a multidimensional definition of partner abuse against women, where severity and frequency are important features of any act against a partner and inclusive of physical, emotional, and sexual acts. Denominators for calculation of response rates need to include refusals and missed patients, and exclusions need to be clearly detailed. The use of research assistants to administer questionnaires maximizes response rates. Prevalence rates should be calculated on women in current relationships, although data should be collected on both current and past relationships to capture the experience of separated and divorced women who have a high rate of partner abuse. It should be clear whether the relationship includes only cohabiters or cohabiters and boyfriends. As outlined clearly in Chapter 13, more information needs to be collected on same-sex relationships.

Finally, continued research in this field is required to answer the following questions. How do we design an IPA educational programme and system change that substantially improves health practitioners' identification rates? Would enquiry about abuse of women presenting with certain problems (e.g. depression or tiredness) or in particular clinics (e.g. sexual health or antenatal) improve disclosure rates? What additional interventions for abused women identified by health professionals will improve their health outcomes? We need research into the effectiveness and appropriateness of universal screening in health care settings or targeting of specific groups (e.g. pregnant women). The impact of increasing abuse enquiry rates by health professionals on management strategies and health outcomes of women who experience violence needs to be examined. Any guidelines on management of domestic violence should be evaluated in terms of health outcomes for women and their children.

Research to improve the response of health professionals and health care systems will require a combination of randomized controlled trials recruiting individual women to specific interventions such as advocacy or counselling, other types of controlled studies using routine data on identification and referral, surveys of health care practice, and qualitative studies of women's experiences and expectations of health systems. Under-investment in domestic violence services internationally is mirrored by the insufficient resources that are available to research the needs of women experiencing IPA and evaluate health care-based interventions. We need national and international studies that take into account cultural and socioeconomic differences, and variation in the structure and delivery of health services. The cross-fertilization of ideas that is visible in this book between doctors, nurses, social workers, psychologists, and other health professionals, health service researchers, policy analysts, and domestic violence service providers, is a strong basis for more robust research and appropriate care for women struggling in the war-zone of IPA.

REFERENCES

1. Davis DA, Thomson MA, Oxman AD, et al. Changing physician performance: a systematic review of the effect of continuing medical education strategies. JAMA 1995; 274(9):700–705.
2. Lohr KN, Carey TS. Assessing 'best evidence': issues in grading the quality of studies for systematic reviews. Jt Comm J Qual Improv 1999; 25:470–479.
3. http://www.cebm.net/levels_of_evidence.asp [accessed 28 July 2004].
4. Rychetnik L, Frommer M, Hawe P, et al. Criteria for evaluating evidence on public health interventions. J Epidemiol Community Health 2002; 56:119–127.
5. Davey SG, Ebrahim S, Frankel S. How policy informs the evidence. BMJ 2001; 322:184–185.
6. Swinkels A, Albarran JW, Means RI, et al. Evidence-based practice in health and social care: where are we now? J Interprof Care 2002; 16:335–347.

Index